D1824689

# Flawless Fitness 2

# Mature Content Warning

Since we live in a very sensitive age, I guess it's my responsibility as an author to announce that this book deals with mature subject matter. It uses colorful swearing along with references to sex, alcohol, and everything else that turns a good party into a *great* party, to illustrate complex fitness techniques.

Why?

Because, I'm into that shit.

# Look Better While Helping Charity

**I will be donating one dollar ($1) from every book sold to help out individuals by donating to a charity of my choosing.** The money will go as and where it's needed - for example the latest tragedy at the time of writing was hurricane Sandy so I'll be donating to causes that help with rebuilding, shelter etc.

Plus, I dig NYC – you can get a pizza slice for a buck, and it's good enough to give you a mouth orgasm. If you believe there is a charity or foundation out there that deserves the money, email me here: **info@flawlessfitnessbook.com** and let me know why.

In the end, wherever the money goes, just know that it will be helping people that need it. I may be a jerk, but I'm not an asshole.

So thanks for buying it, you're fucking awesome.

# Copyright & Other Legal Shit

Flawless Fitness 2
First Digital Edition (V 1.0) was published, May 19 2012
First Hardcover was published late 2012 or early 2013; I wish I knew
the exact date, but I had to send in this final draft and twiddle my
thumbs while I waited for Amazon to give it a green light. Once it
did, it finally went on sale.

Published under: Flawless Fitness Media
(**www.flawlessfitnessmedia.com**)
ISBN-13: 978-1477530627

**This book is designed to be read cover-to-cover and therefore,
the index/contents are listed at the end.**

If you're interested in training under my guidance, then go here:
**http://www.flawlessfitnessbook.com/e-training-sales.html**

Serious inquiries only. Once you fill out your information, I will
send you a series of questions that you must answer in as much
detail as possible. If you're a good match for E-Training, I'll take you
on board and get you some serious results.

On the other hand, if you don't need me to hold your hand every
stop of the way, and just need a full-fledged 12 week fitness program
customized and created just for you, check out my Personal Body
Blueprint here: **http://flawlessfitnessbook.com/fitness-
blueprint.html**

# Dedicated To...

... My Family, Best Friends, Good Friends, Bros, Random Acquaintances, Ex's, Fellow Bloggers, Fellow Haters, MILFS, Hotties I've Spanked, Hotties That've Spanked Me, Hotties That Want To Spank Me, Future Unknown Woman Of My Sexy Offspring(s) And Most Importantly, My Loyal Readers And Customers...

This Book Will Add Life To Your Years, While Adding Years To Your Life (And If It Doesn't, You Probably Read It Wrong!)

- Sahil M (a.k.a "FitJerk")

# Foreword by a handsome dude from Sweden

*"I have been impressed with the urgency of doing. Knowing is not enough; we must apply. Being willing is not enough; we must do."* - *Leonardo da Vinci*

Why would you possibly be interested in a book by FitJerk? After all, there are dozens of "nice" people out there who are careful not to offend, stay politically correct, avoid stepping on anyone's toes and have effective training methods of their own... so why bother listening to a man with a colorful vocabulary and an intense personality?

Because FJ is a guy who realizes that all the scientific studies, theoretical knowledge, and fitness programs are worthless unless the most important factor is present - **doing work.**

You want fat loss? Sure, I can personally get you a big pile of research papers, showing which methods work best in a clinical setting. You want to add lean, sexy mass to your frame? No problem, I probably know 50 different training templates that could give you exactly that.

Then why is it, despite the enormous and constantly increasing number of effective programs, that people just can't seem to get the body they've always dreamed of? Why is it that despite hundreds of TV shows, fitness magazines and personal trainers, people still can't look themselves in the mirror and smile at what they are seeing?

Because they fail to grasp the fundamentals of doing work and lack motivation, which is what makes ANY training or dieting program successful - in the short or long term.

This is when you might need a certain "Jerk" to jump-start the process for you, because if you don't put in the work, then it's all just an illusion. Nothing but a pipe-dream.

FJ's words are as powerful as they are hilarious; they will inspire you to want to change your body; improve your health; look sexy and rip your shirt off at the beach. Instead of hand holding, sometimes you just need someone who'll never ever let you give up. He doesn't care about your feelings, nor does he pay much attention to your excuses.

He is the one who will make sure you are working hard even when motivation starts to fade. This man will always tell you what you need, even if it's not necessarily what you want. I've come to realize that he cares for one thing, and one thing only - your results.

This book will teach you the theoretical facts and principles of fat loss, the best resistance training methods and most importantly, it'll teach you how to wake up every day and strive for excellence, not the norm.

If you need to get your ass kicked from time to time (and trust me, we all do) – then this is the perfect book for you, written by the perfect man. Congratulations for taking the first step, now turn the page and start doing some work. You will not regret it.

See you at the beach!

Dr. Bojan Kostevski
**www.lift-heavy.com**

# An Independent Panel Of Experts Have Deemed This Book To Be...

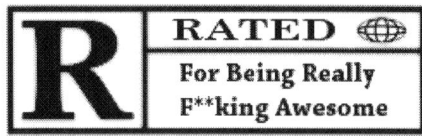

"When FJ first told me he was coming out with a new book I couldn't help but bust out a couple of fist pumps. Granted, I was in a local coffee shop and accidentally punched a cute lady passing by in the jaw, but hey, she shouldn't have been walking there! I digress. The main reason I'm excited FJ decided to publish a new book is because I know he provides quality, science-based information. Not only is FJ an incredible source of info but his passion for helping others achieve their own training goals is second to none. If you truly want to better yourself and learn from one of the smartest guys in the industry, I strong believe that investing in FJ's book is a wise decision – you won't be disappointed!"

Jordan Syatt

**www.syattfitness.com**

"I have known the FJ for quite a few years now. One of the reasons he's one of my favorite writers is his frank and direct advice. He doesn't sugar coat or waste time, he gets right to the point. If you want results, his methods are what you need to follow. He'll take the best research in the field, break it down and formulate to his own brand of magic. His methods are quick, efficient and so easy to follow that you deserve to be called an idiot if this doesn't work for you!"

Kris R

**www.selfrecoverynow.com**

"Combine science, hilarity and experience with a dose of tough love, and what do you get? The Fittest Jerk of them all. FJ has about as many reps with real world clients as he does with lifting. Just check out some of his kickass client transformations and testimonials. Quit relying on broscience, myths, and programs that have you panting hard while leaving you flabby still. FJ will get you in the best shape of your life while you actually have fun in the process."

Dick Talens, Co-Founder Of Fitocracy
**www.fitocracy.com**

"If I had to describe Fitjerk, one word simply wouldn't do. FJ is a mix between a lion, Jiminy Cricket and the big brother you never had. He'll get up in your face and keep you from letting your excuses keep you from your goals while also giving you all the tools you'll need to be successful (with a healthy dose of tough love thrown in for pizazz). FJ also walks the walk, so rest assured that your results are in good hands."

Roger Lawson II
**www.roglawfitness.com**

"Dear FJ,

I have to tell you... being a gymnast for 13 years had given me an 'I know everything' kind of attitude in regards to fitness. I mean, this sport is very physically demanding so I had no reason to accept fitness advice from others. However, after reading Flawless Fitness I have had my brain completely re-wired! Your eBook has totally opened me up to all sorts of new techniques and principals that have helped me progress at a rate that I have never experienced before!

I strongly recommend this book to anyone who is serious about reaching their fitness goals or taking their current workout to the next level. I love how you go into so much detail in regards to optimum work out times which help you effectively reach your goals faster than, say... a guy who spends 3-4 hours in a gym but is not working out properly.

I have been using what I've learned in the book for the past 3 weeks now and without a doubt... I have reached a whole new level in muscular strength and definition which would not have been possible without your eBook."
Steven Sugrim, lead bass player for Dreamers
**www.dreamerswtf.com**

"If there is anyone who tells it like it is without being around the bush, it is the FitJerk. He has this unique combination of providing useful information while telling you to man up (or woman up). His material is like taking a shot of espresso while getting punched in the face at the same time. Yeah it's weird, but it works. At first when reading FJ's work, you will feel your ego being tossed around like a ping pong ball.

Stick with the pain, don't shut this out. He might sound like he is being harsh, but this guy honestly cares about changing people's lives. He wants to see you let go of your limiting beliefs and become the ultimate human being. He wants you to walk around with your head up high while feeling highly confident about yourself. I approve FJ as being a positive influence to the masses. Much respect."
Jon Fernandes
**www.jonfernandes.com**

"The fitness industry is saturated with feel-good, motivational, and up-beat personalities that never hesitate to give you a pat on the back. Logging onto FitJerk's site is like a swift kick to the face. Albeit, a much needed and refreshing one.
FJ provides a stark contrast to the status quot by fostering a zero nonsense, straight to the point approach that oozes passion. RESULTS, by the most effective and unique methods possible is what comes to mind when trying to describe what he does.

Ask any of his clients, and they will tell you there were no hugs or "koombaya's" to be had, but the jaw dropping results speak for themselves. His unique background allows for an approach unlike most. Not only do his clients get transformed physically, but their mental state strengthens exponentially. I myself have gained considerable strength in my own mindset through FJ's quality articles and posts.

He will continue to influence many of my decisions as a fitness professional, as well as countless others in the industry. Oh yeah. He also holds the Canadian National Deadlift Record in his weight class. So you know he walks the walk."
Josh Hamilton, Personal Trainer
**www.joshhamiltonfitness.com**

# What's New?

More like, what isn't new? This was supposed to be the 2nd edition to my original book, which in hindsight was so-so, but by the time I was half way through the process, I realized that too much was re-written and added. Therefore it was time for me to make an executive decision, and so I said, "Screw the new edition, it's time to release a sequel!"

And so I did. You'll find that my sequel is actually be epic, unlike 90% of the movies that come out of Hollywood.

If you're a first time customer of the Flawless Fitness Book, then you may skip this section if you wish. But if you're an original book holder then boy oh boy, do I have a few surprises for you. First things first, know that the focus of this book has changed. My earlier product was more of an "all-rounder". It covered nutrition, muscle gains, workout planning and had a heavy emphasis on optimizing your daily energy. This book will cover those topics as well, but this time around my aim was focused like a death ray towards one target: fat loss.

I noticed that most people who purchased the earlier versions wanted to get as lean as possible and generally look more awesome without clothes on. Therefore, I figured it was time to release something that did fat loss with high efficiency.

You're about to discover advanced fat loss tactics such as weekly carbohydrate cycling, visiting the "dark" side of supplementation with potent substances (if you choose to use them), a breakdown of the Paleo diet, a look at intermittent fasting, food substitutes and shit loads more. I threw away the decision to be ethical in order to provide you with the best information on fat loss.

Later on when we put together your plan, you can choose whether to use all the tools available or just the ones that fit your lifestyle , your budget or your values - whatever they happen to be. As far as I'm concerned, absolutely nothing was held back.

While this book is much more advanced, you may still use all the advice and workout principals from the first book, only now you have even more options. It's one of the perks of being an early adopter of my work (unlike being an early adopter of say, Apple™ products).

For the new customers who, for some reason are still reading along, know that I have taken the best from the past, and the best from the present to produce something that will deliver stellar results for your future. I used to have a 6 pack by doing what I used to do... now I pretty much have an 8 pack. This means you'll be getting tips and techniques that are nothing but the best of the best. Evolution is a beautiful thing.

# How To Use This Book

Ok, so you bought the book and are eager to start, awesome! But first, forget EVERYTHING! That's right, forget anything and everything you know or think you know about fitness or fat loss and read this book with an open mind. If you do this, your success rate will skyrocket. I spent a lot of time and energy writing these stack of pages, so the last thing we both need is your past knowledge conflicting with what I'm trying to teach you.

Also, let me assure you that this book has everything you need, but you *must always* come back to it. Think of it as a user's manual that your body never came with. God forgot, so now I'm doing his work. I feel like a saint. SaintJerkus, to be exact.

I also don't want you to skim through this literary beast, hopping around from section to section for your next information fix. I suggest you read this book from cover to cover because I have structured everything in a specific way. That's why the table of contents is at the *end*. (No, you don't have to go look – trust me it's there.)

This structure is going to get you motivated and most importantly, *keep* you motivated. It will also show you what to do and what *not* to do. So follow my lead, as I am about to show you some really kick-ass techniques that will blow you away, all of which I personally use to keep my body in peak shape year-round!

I highly recommend that you have a printed version of this book. This way, you can toss it in your gym or school bag and always have the information at hand. I have attached blank pages at the end so that you may have space to record your progress along the way.

Remember, you *must* write down the progress you are making. It is a proven fact that you are 80% more likely to achieve your goal and stick to it if you write it down.

That is how powerful this stuff is. Now that you know this, put it to good use.

Also, take a 'before' shot of yourself in as little clothing as possible. Do it right now... strip I say!

Make sure you take it in an environment which you can replicate in the future, because you should be taking pictures weekly. Nothing will get you motivated like seeing your body change on a weekly basis right in front of your eyes. It's freaky, it's awesome and it should be done.

# "Why Do They Call You A 'Jerk', Dude?"

While this little section isn't what I'd call "mandatory reading", I figured it was important to include a mini history lesson since there are way too many misconceptions about why the hell I'm called what I am. First things first, I did not randomly wake up one day and say, "hey I know, I should call myself... FitJerk. Yeah, that sounds highly desirable and marketable!"

No, the name actually came from a very early book customer. It was a lady (god bless her). She bought it, read it and then fired an email asking for some further guidance. This was no problem, so I banged out a massive email and made sure I over-delivered in the response. She was happy with everything but there was one problem... no action was being taken. I didn't get it. I had made her a kick-ass workout plan, she knew how to go about it, she bought the required groceries and supplements but she just wouldn't get *moving*.

Oh the frustration! On top of that she kept emailing me, asking questions which would be auto-answered if she just got her hands dirty. Questions such as:

"How do I know that there is lactic acid buildup in my muscles?"

"Uhm... you'll feel a burning sensation and you can't complete a full rep. By the way have you actually started the plan yet? It's much easier to experience this sensation than talk about it."

"No, not yet"

Frustration would have been considered an understatement at that point. So that was it, I knew it was time to lay the verbal smack down, otherwise she'd just keep consuming a mind-bending amount of information and not do jack all with it. So off I went, to send her a little reality check.

See, unlike most authors, I like to follow up and make sure that the info people paid good money for is being applied. After this "reality check" she responded by saying, "I guess I needed to hear that, so thanks, I think. Though I have to say that you're a bit of a jerk... although a fit one. I'll start the plan tomorrow, promise."

Hmm, a "fit jerk"? After all I did for her, how dare she call me such things! But as the minutes flew by, the words just grew on me. A fit jerk... somehow those two words just make sense. So after ignoring the advice of my peers (they thought the name was a terrible idea), I thought to myself, *"Hmm, I might as well use a name that embodies what I stand for, that way people know what to expect."* So yes, I'm a jerk at times. But it's for a good reason. I've found there are three major ways to motivate someone...

Hand holding, Ass kissing or Ass kicking.

The latter is just more efficient. But I'm far from an asshole. It's an important distinction you need to keep in mind.

And here's the nugget of wisdom I want you to focus on as you read along: **Knowledge isn't power unless applied**. While I got nuthin' but love for my customers and clients, I don't take in-action lightly. This book isn't some self-help spiritual feel-good shit. It's meant to change your life, if you let it.

# Ground Zero: Upgrading Your Crappy Brain OS* (Mentality)

*OS – noun: Short for Operating System such as Windows or OSX*

# The Blame Game

At this point I'm supposed to tell you that it's not your fault. You shouldn't blame yourself or beat yourself up for the state that you are in, and instead point the finger elsewhere. Blame the government, the farmers or whatever other nonsense most fitness "gurus" regurgitate out of their stinkin' mouths. Sometimes I wonder if they have the slightest grasp of reality.

Now let me back up for a second. Are there "bad guys" out there who put high fructose corn syrup (which isn't that bad), MSG, hormones and other garbage in your food? Yes. Are there greedy pigs who only care about profit margins rather than the state of your health? Yes. But are they forcing you to eat what they produce? Hell no. In the end, while making healthier choices is becoming slightly inconvenient, it has not by any stretch of the imagination, become impossible.

So I really don't have to tell you who's "fault" it is. I think you know exactly which decisions you've made in your past that are responsible for your current physical state. If you sit down and think about it logically, you can track your physical decline from the sexy, to the not so sexy to your present condition... and I'll be the first to tell you, that this truly is a hard pill to swallow.

But this is why you're here. You didn't pay money for this book to read nice fluffy words that will cushion the blow of my verbal spank on your ass. Nor is it my intention to provide a state of mental bliss where everything will be dandy. You paid money to change your life around and that's something which needs to be shocked into you.

Owning and taking responsibility for your actions is the first step towards change. No one else cares about your success more than you do.

In fact, most people would rather see you fail because they don't have the balls to step up and take control of their lives. It bugs them when others achieve something they could only dream about. Again, I'm not saying that everyone is out to "get" you, but when you really think about it, you are the only one that is in control of your life... or at least you will be, by the time I'm through with you.

Take a moment and accept the reality of your situation. While at first it might feel a bit saddening, it should equally feel empowering to know that what you did can be undone because you have the power to take action. It's in your hands. I will be showing you the doors of opportunity but I will not be dragging you through them. That's your job - for now, and until you hit your death bed.

# Mental Masturbation

There are many weight loss books that focus on the mental aspect of things, but the problem is that they end up reading like fruity self- help pieces of hilarity instead of providing any solid advice. They tell you to regurgitate beliefs, talk about positivity and suggest you meditate for 2 hours a day... *hummmmmmm*. A few books even throw in some NLP (neuro linguistic programming) techniques and practically brainwash you into a delusional confidence exuding werido.

I call this Mental Masturbation. There is a difference between the mind/body connection and outright fruitcake tendencies. I think the reason they focus on these topics so hardcore is so that when you realize their methods don't work, you'll still be an optimistic sheep, carry on with an unsatisfying life, not see results and still not lay blame on the author.

Fuck that. If something didn't work, you have every right to be pissed off. Getting angry every now and then is ok. As a human, you need to experience the wide range of emotions that were handed down to you by your ancestors. Just don't do anything idiotic when you're angry... feeling emotions and taking actions are two different things, even *if* emotions do help motivate those actions. It's your job to decide what's right and what's wrong.

However, not all of this mental hoopla is useless. I do follow "basic mental masturbation" on a daily basis because no one likes a negative, self-victimizing prick. I might be a jerk, but ask anyone that knows me - I'm a blast to be around. I make sure I'm the life of the party and this has gotten me far in life. Here are some of the basic things I practice:

Tell negative people to screw off, and never return.

When I encounter someone who is a life drain, they get the boot. Either literally or I cease to communicate and/or contact them any further. Their negativity is just not worth my time. Eliminate any and all negative people in your life right now and don't let any more of these life suckers enter. Some people will be easier to eliminate than others, but you have to do this. Oh, and just so were clear, "eliminating" a person from your life does not mean eliminating them from the world... that's not nice, even if it may be well justified.

Have some core values

"Give advice only to those who seek it..."
"Go after what you want until you get it..."
"Don't accept bullshit from others..."

Can you guess what those statements are? They're 3 of my 10 core values that I have. My set of values is my personal code. It keeps me on track and helps me move forward while avoiding circumstances that aren't in my best interest or just don't sit well with me. You can make up your own set of core values. I don't care what they are, just make sure to be honest and live by them day in and day out.

For example, if there is a person I don't really like but they happen to come up to me and genuinely ask for health & fitness advice... I'll give it to them. Why? It's just one of my values; it's what I do. On the contrary, if I hear someone bitching and moaning about how they're out of shape and can't change because of some lame excuse, then I won't help them. In fact I'll probably bust their balls. Why? Because that's who I am. It might not be who you are, so practice your values accordingly. If you are doing something and it feels "wrong," then chances are you are not living in alignment with your values. Define them, live by them and you'll truly live free.

Do what you can to relax and or enjoy things on a daily basis.

It's not necessary to get into a lotus pose and meditate for an hour (though basic meditative breathing is something that helps). There are other methods which you can use to relax and reduce stress. If it means taking a bubble bath with your favorite plastic boat toy, then screw it, take the damn bath. If you like reading dirty romance novels in the candle light, I say go for it.

Do what you need to do to chill out at least twice a day. I usually relax about 3-4 times a day. It keeps me sane and functioning, especially considering the hair-ripping emails I often get. But hey, I reply to each and every one. I might be more awesome than most people, but I'm not too big to respond back to a genuine email, or a tweet, or a facebook comment. (tweet me here: twitter.com/fitjerk and bookface me here: facebook.com/fitjerk.fanpage)

# The Only Belief You'll Ever Need

I often deal with people with low morale or the self- esteem of a homeless person who extinguished his supply of crack. Sure enough, one common denominator that these people have is the lack of beliefs in this world. So I tell them that there is just one thing they need to believe in, and that is: "**you can achieve anything you put your mind to.**"

That's it, that's all you'll ever need. But the hard part is to actually internalize this belief. The most powerful way to do this is through proof and experience. For example: If horribleness constantly happens to someone, they'll usually cultivate a belief that they are unlucky... and will go through life not trying and giving up because hey, it's not their fault, their just unlucky right? Absolute nonsense. But it's not hard to see the power life experience has had on them. So how do you believe in something you don't have proof of? Well, you start with small tasks.

Think of a small task that you never bothered to try because you thought you lacked the skills or weren't good enough. Then attempt that task till you succeed. It could be anything from climbing a tree to baking a cake. Once you accomplish it, realize that you succeeded because you put your mind to it - not because you got lucky or because god answered your prayers.

After that, tackle a bigger challenge and then an even bigger one, till that shit snowballs and you're living the life you want... while having the body to match. Get what I'm saying? Good. Now get in that kitchen and go bake that cake, I'm starving.

# A Potent Shot Of Motivation

I have included this piece so that you can come back and re-motivate yourself on days you go off-track. You see, there are a lot of people who write fitness books, some are good and some are (let's be honest) pure crap. I know because I've pretty much read them all. But if you take a look at their overall reader base, I bet only about 10-20% of them actually put the information to good use.

Maybe even less!

They buy the information, they look, they try, then give up and get on with the same old miserable life that they were living before. Pathetic. Absolutely NO change takes place. The worst part is that the authors don't care. Why should they? They made their money and are enjoying life. (Or went broke and are now spending the remainder of their time in a shed, accompanied by their right hand... or left if they're feeling rather adventurous on that day.)

Well, I believe that the customer who bought that book is partially to blame for their lack of commitment, but the author is partially to blame also.

WHY?

Well, it's easy to slap together a book with workouts in it... no big deal. In fact, I can slap one up in a WEEK with all the information I have in my head, but instead I want to add real value to your life.

This is where I am hoping to close the gap. It is human nature to get distracted, but that's ok, we are going to cheat it together. It's completely normal for you to go off track once in a while, I do it too. But just because you had a little slip, does not mean you cannot get back on track.

One main reason is that right now you have my book, and I will help keep your 'train' of will-power on that track to success. The information in here will really hits home for you.

I am basically going to tell you WHY you need to keep going, and stick to your plan. Answer the following question without using a calculator or doing any math in your head, just guess:

How many days do you get on this planet? (From the time you are born till the time you die)

Thousands
Tens of thousands
Hundreds of thousands
Millions

Did you make a guess? Good.

Head on to the next page for the shocking answer...

The answer is roughly 29,000 days. Even if you live to be 100 years old, that's only 36,500 days.

Now out of those days, think about how many have already been used up. If you are in your 30s, then it's safe to assume that around 1/3 of your days are history. So if 1/3 of the 29,000 days you get on this planet have been used up, you now have 19,430 days left.

Ok, now out of 19,430 days, how many are left to enjoy life to the fullest? Because let's face it, sitting in a retirement home with an oxygen machine hooked up to you while you play bingo isn't living life... or maybe it is?

The truth is that without doing any further math, the simple answer is that you do NOT have that much time. A hard pill to swallow? Better believe it!

So doesn't it make sense that you do everything in your power to enhance every day of your life? Doesn't it make sense that you take action RIGHT NOW and make a commitment to live everyday to the fullest?

Shit, it sure does to me. And the great thing is, if you are in shape you can actually re-claim some of those days you think you have lost. I have seen people who have been physically active and the effect it has had on their lives. This change can happen in as little as 60 days!

I have seen 55 year old men that look like they are in their late 30's. I have seen grandmothers that look so good, they could model in Victoria's Secret catalogues (no joke!) I can keep going with examples but you get the point. The facts are obvious - taking care of your body will give you a more enjoyable life no matter what you do. So ask yourself... isn't that worth spending some time and hard work on?

The answer should be a resounding, "Fuck Yes!"

# Here's The Real Secret To Success!

*"Motivation is what gets you started, habit is what keeps you going" -*
*Jim Ryun*

$W$hat I am about to tell you, will probably be the most important thing you have ever read. This secret will keep you on track, make you get off your ass and do something to change your body into a state that it DESERVES to be in. Do you want to know why some people in life are considered winners and get the results they want while others don't?

Before I give you the answer, know that these 'winners' are not always smarter than you, in fact most of them are just as lazy as you are!

The answer is that these winners (or achievers) in life, know how to implement a habit quicker and more efficiently than non-achievers. Seems simple, but it is much harder to do than it sounds. Actually, truth be told it's quite the bitch. I know because I constantly see people walking through life in zombie mode.

They can't seem to get out of this dull trance which consumes them. They won't listen to what others are trying to tell them, even if it's for their own good! They are also afraid of change, because breaking their normal routine will require some extra work in the beginning.

Well screw that, because if you want results (and I know you do) then you are going to have to put in some work to implement new habits, but most importantly, BREAK out of bad ones! The way I implement a habit is first I look at what I want to accomplish. It can be *any* goal. In this case, let's take my old goal so that you can relate. I used to be VERY light - underweight for my height. I decided that I wanted to get from 110 to 140 lbs. Now 140 lbs is still light, but I do power tumbling and acrobatics so I still need to be limber and agile.

The next thing is to formulate a plan. I acquired the knowledge I needed, then I made a routine (work out for one hour, 4 days a week while implementing a proper eating lifestyle) and accepted this as my daily part of life.

The final and most important thing I did was, divert my focus AWAY from the outcome and instead made sure to follow my plan no matter what, even in less ideal and unlikely conditions. It did not matter if it rained, snowed, hailed or if I had to walk, drive, or rely on public transportation. I made sure I went 4 days a week and followed my eating habits with no exceptions. You have to trust the plan that you have set (or the plan your coach has set) and know that it will guide you to your destination.

I won't lie. The first week was a bit difficult because my body was not used to training 4 days a week while consuming so much food. Working out while being tired was also pretty tough. See, when you are initially implementing a plan, your mind always focuses on the tedious road that lies ahead because the beginning seems hard. I still remember the day I started my routine and thinking: "woah... another 3-4 months of THIS?! This shit is gona take forever!"

But a funny thing happened. After about 3 weeks, the routine became natural and I went into autopilot. I didn't even have to think about eating so much... I just did it. I never had to force myself to hit the gym, every night I just went.

Soon my body just craved it, it became enjoyable and I knew that if I skipped a day, I would feel like crap. Currently I'm at about 140lbs with 5-6% body fat.

So to recap, I realized that my initial bitching was too outcome oriented. If you are always outcome-focused you are never going to get results because the road you must travel may seem long. Focus on what you have to do right NOW so that you will end up where you want. If you drive across the country, you can't see your destination... you can only see about 50 feet of road in front, which your headlights are illuminating. But you keep driving. Why? Because you know without a doubt that if you keep heading the right direction, you'll eventually get there.

Fitness works in the exact same manner. Now that you know this, just focus on sticking to your habit and gauge your success based on the question: "Did I stick to my habit today?" and not "Why am I not at my (X) weight yet?!"

# Happy Memory

While trainers always try their best to make sure that their clients get the best technical advice possible, most hardly take the time to explain the psychological tools that need to go hand in hand with the given plan to make sure it "sticks." To me, increasing the stick ratio of a program is far more important than seeing constant weekly improvements.

Why?

Well, because if a client can be consistent, then their future improvements in terms of body composition and strength is virtually guaranteed. It might take slightly longer than I want, but I know beyond a shadow of a doubt that it will come. If a client quits however, it's a sure sign that seeing any form of improvement is a pipe dream. Kind of like my chances of hooking up with Scarlette Johanson. Tear.

Besides motivation, one easy way to increase the "stick ratio" is to put yourself into a happy state, both mentally and physically, while performing actions that relate to your fitness plan. For example, I've found that 99.9% of the population absolutely loathes keeping their daily meal logs up to date. People sit down at their computers or in front of their journal and grumble before putting the pen to paper or keyboard to computer. These people are essentially linking their sad/unhappy state to their actions.

So now, every time they feel sad or unhappy in the future, it will bring back the memories of them updating their meal plan journals. Attaching a negative emotion to an action that's supposed to help you achieve your goals is a horrible fucking idea. Even if you manage to keep your journal up to date, the mere action of doing so will mentally exhaust you.

Why do you think most students feel like sleeping when it's time to study, yet they can pull all-nighters playing video games every day of the week? (Hint: they've linked happy emotions to video games and negative emotions to edjumacation!)

The solution is to "fake" yourself into feeling happy. Put on a big ass synthetic smile, play music that pumps you up, and even yell "I feel awesome, because I am awesome!" while beating your chest if you have to. Do whatever it takes to change your physiology so that it puts you in a more positive state. Then and only then, proceed by taking actions which are necessary to achieve your goals. What you'll be doing is linking a positive state (happy/excited) to a physical action (working out and/or updating your meal plan.)

If at this point you're chuckling at the ridiculousness of what I wrote in the last two paragraphs, **then it's because you still have no idea as to how obnoxiously powerful this little technique can be.** You've got to give it a shot. Oh in case you're not aware, it can be applied to almost any area of your life where actions that lead to improvement are necessary.

**Why It Works**

Without getting too technical, the basic principal is that your memory is highly state dependent. When you're happy, you'll have an easier time remembering other times when you were happy. When you're pissed off, you'll have an easier time remembering other times when you were pissed off.

Ever notice that when you're out partying, you have an easier time recalling other times you were partying and have plenty of awesome drunk stories to tell your friends? Yeah, that ain't the booze, it's the concept of state dependent memory working. Though, the booze does change your physiology (you feel relaxed and happy) which obviously facilitates this happy memory recall. Until of course, you drink so much that memory recall turns into memory loss. But that's a different topic all together.

The same is true when you're pissed. Let's say you get into a fight with your significant other - notice how easy it is to recall other times when they pissed you off. You'll likely remember the date, the reason, the location along with a shit load of other details which you can use as verbal ammo.

This concept explains the bizarre love which people have when it comes to lifting weights. Logically, there is nothing pleasurable about lifting weights at all. It's heavy as hell, it makes you sweat, it's painful, it requires a tremendous amount of mental focus, it makes you extremely sore, it makes you hungry and results don't come instantly. So why do people like me, love lifting? It's because we always put ourselves in such a positive state before we do. I listen to good music, pump myself up by looking in the mirror, put on a happy face and try and compete with my workout partner. I've attached those positive emotions to the physical action of lifting for so long, that now the action itself has become pleasurable... even though physically, it's anything but.

*As you read through the book, you might be wondering why I listed my references chapter by chapter and therefore, might be inclined to email me saying, "that's not how it's done". But please don't bother. This is more efficient, and if you don't think so, too bad. My book, my method. There are no set ways of doing things. Rules exist so you know when to break them. Now, let us focus on something more important...*

# Chapter 1: Put Down The Cupcake, And Lets Get Started

# The Term "Ripped"

Let me clarify this little word since it's the basis of my book.
Everything you are about to read revolves around getting you
"ripped". For the savvy individuals who have active social lives and
are up to date on the hip lingo, you probably know what I'm talking
about. In that case, skip this section and move along.

But for those of you who are dazed and confused, and feel left out...
let me hold your hand and explain. Looking ripped basically means
that you possess a body that is chiseled, lean, sexy, hot etc. Here is
my official definition:

**Ripped** *[ript] –adjective,*
*A human body that has an attractive amount of lean muscle tissue*
*along with a fat percentage of 10% or lower.* Example: *"Holy shit*
*dude, that guy is so ripped you can see all of his abs! If I were a*
*woman, I'd totally do him right now. But I'm not. Seriously."*

Now, I understand that not everyone wants a body fat percentage of
10% or lower. Some are just looking to be "healthy". And those
individuals are what I like to call, "under-achievers". Stop aiming for
mediocracy, it's pathetic. By the end of this book you will have, in
your very hands, the perfect road map to achieve 10% or lower body
fat. So why wouldn't you? This goes for men and women, by the
way.

And just in case you need more convincing as to why you should
strive for a body that is lean and mean, consider a recent study[1-1]
published in *Military Medicine* which compared how body fat levels
affects the performance of soldiers. They took two groups of
soldiers, one at < 18% body fat and the others at 18%+ body fat.

The results were unsurprising, to say the least: *"**Results showed group 1: < 18% BF performed significantly better on 7 of the 10 fitness tests. In Soldiers with similar amounts of FFM, Soldiers with less body fat had improved aerobic and anaerobic capacity and increased muscular strength.**"* In layman's terms, the lean soldiers were stronger *and* had better cardio.

That's not saying that heavy individuals aren't strong, (I'm sure you've seen fat powerlifters move enormous weight) but in the army and in the real world, lifting heavy stuff just once isn't enough. You need a balance of endurance, strength and sex appeal. Low body fat levels help you achieve all three.

Another thing to keep in mind is the number on the scale. There have been countless occasions where E-Training clients email me with massive amounts of confusion saying *"FJ, I stepped on the scale this week and I'm no lighter! I feel so discouraged, all that hard work ... oh and on a side note, my pants don't fit me anymore. I need to buy like a whole new set of shorts. What gives?!"* Actual emails are much longer but that's the jist of it.

So understand that if your net weight doesn't change much, there is no reason to freak out and send me a three page long essay. What the mirror tells you is far more important. In fact, it's the ultimate truth! When you're walking down the beach, no one gives a shit whether you're 160lbs or 155lbs, so stop stressing over the number.

Muscle is denser then fat, and our goal is to put on more of the former and burn down more of the latter. Doing this will result in the lean and sexy physique that will turn heads so fast that people's head will snap in your direction. Take my word for it, and of those whom I've caused involuntary neck sprain by walking shirtless down the beach.

# How To Set And Achieve Goals

Whether you want to admit it or not, achieving goals is an art. It takes practice, repetition and constant effort to get good at aiming at a target, then hitting it with ridiculous precision. Those that are good at achieving goals have usually developed their own system over the many years of basking in success, learning from failures, and basically, not being losers. No one is born knowing how to achieve a specific outcome.

What's funny is that 90% of people will disagree with that statement. But just remember that those are the same morons who can't seem to accomplish anything in the first place. So don't fall for their bullshit. Would you rather do what 90% of people are doing, or the 10% that are living the life you want to live? Thought so.

Here's another interesting fact: While no one is born knowing how to achieve an outcome, it seems nearly everyone is highly potent at dreaming up specific goals and plans that will ultimately get them to where they want to be. Basically, we humans have no problem finding targets, but when it's time to take action, we absolutely suck.

I mean honestly, just look around you. How many people in your social circle have said that they want to achieve something big or significant? And have any of them actually done so? My guess is not many.

You see, losers don't know how to walk the talk, so they just keep on talking.

This is also the reason why I screen potential E-Training prospects before I take them on as clients. I want mental winners from the start! I mean sure, who the hell doesn't want to lose weight and look great?

Everyone has a goal, but not everyone is committed to taking action and doing what is necessary to transform goals from a mere dream to reality.

So if you have a massive list of goals that you've made in the past but have yet to follow through any of them, I'm going to break down my simple 4 step process that is virtually bullet-proof. It not only works, but it works every time... all you have to do is not screw around and implement it.

## 1. Pick An Attainable Goal

If you're learning to play the guitar, then you might have goals of becoming a rock legend one day. If you're a huge nerd that battles evil warlords on your computer, than you might one day want to become a seductive "player" that bangs 5 strippers every week. All admirable goals, but the probability of you attaining them is so low, you have a better chance of catching lightning by running around in the rain with a spoon up your ass. There is a fine line between dreaming big, and dreaming ridiculous.

So, pick an attainable goal – whatever that means for you. Look in the mirror and think about what you can realistically achieve. Then after you've achieved it, you can ALWAYS go after a more ambitious goal. For me, being obnoxiously good looking was a very attainable goal since I was already a handsome chap to begin with. It wasn't much of a stretch, get what I'm saying?

And if you insist on dreaming big right now, then small chunk that dream into a few pieces and make one of those pieces your attainable goal. So, let's say you want to own a mansion. Well a mansion costs millions of dollars, which you'll have to make, and the only way to make millions is to sell lots of awesome shit to a shit load of people. So maybe your goal can be finding awesome shit to sell, or to find a market big and rich enough that will buy the shit you'll want to sell. Does that shit make sense? Good shit!

Once you have this goal, write it down using a sharpie and stick that piece of glory on your wall. While you're at it, remove everything else from your wall (like your stupid Justin Bieber poster) that will distract you from viewing your goal on a daily basis. This piece of paper should be the focal point in your room, no exceptions.

## 2. Pick A Deadline... Now Reduce It By 30%

This second step is simple when stated on paper (or on screen), but hard to follow through as it has a tendency to mentally violate people's brain in naughty ways. You might think you want to achieve your goal by a certain point but the truth of the matter is, a 1/3 of that time you've set for yourself is simply a waste. It's a buffer zone which you don't need. There is a phenomenon called the Parkinson's Law which states the following: **Work expands to fill the time available for its completion.**

Basically, it means that whatever deadline you've set up for yourself, there's a very good chance that that's the exact amount of time it will take for you to achieve your goal... regardless of how much work there is to be done. If you were ever a college student, you've experienced this phenomenon when professors turn into major assholes and won't extend the due date of a paper when you've got a million things going on. Yet somehow, most people manage to hand that damn paper in on time, only to wonder a day later how they pulled off the impossible. Well, it's Parkinson's Law at work. The more time you give yourself, the more work your brain will come up with to fill that gap of time.

So if you want to be deadly effective at achieving goals, set a deadline, then reduce it by thirty percent, or even *fifty percent* if you really want to be an over-achiever. I guarantee you'll have enough time to get it done. Your brain will find a way, mainly by eliminating useless tasks. One of the brilliant ideas that I dawned upon, was the use of virtual assistants (or any type of paid assistant) to do part of the research for me.

This allowed me to focus on what I do best – write content that is edgy, over the top, and gives you a swift kick in the ass.

### 3. Small Chunk And Make A Daily Action Plan

Now that you have your goal and your timeline, small chunk it down like a 2-bite brownie until you have daily action steps which you can take. As an example, to earn $1 million per year, you need to be making $2,778 per day. So your daily action plan is to find a way to earn $2,778. Once you can do that consistently every day, you'll have your million by the end of the year.

I understand your goals may not be based on monetary gains, which is expected since you *are* reading a fitness book. Just make sure your daily action steps can be backtracked accurately so that it leads to your original goal. Taking the example I used above, if you multiply $2,778 by 365 you get $1,013,970. So you know that shit works.

After you have your daily action plan with all the necessary steps, focus on that plan and that plan only. Have tunnel vision. Don't add huge ass things to your to-do list. If you focus on what you have to do on a daily basis, the rest of the year will take care of itself. Don't worry about checking your bank balance or your weight every gosh darn day. As long as you're following your daily plan, your bank account, your body weight or whatever goal you've set for yourself, *will* be achieved. You just have to trust the process.

### 4. Set Up A Reward And A Punishment

For most people, the mere fact of achieving a goal will be a reward in an of itself. For example, if a lonely person's goal was to get a hot girlfriend/boyfriend, then the fact that they could be basking in the afterglow of a hot bang session is quite the reward. Or if someone's goal was to finally bench-press 2x their body weight, then the fact that they'll be "high" from all the adrenaline pumping through their body, along with a feeling of accomplishment will be one helluva reward.

But why not take it a step further? Who said you have to settle for the goal itself? Write down a reward under your goal from step 1. It could be a material possession (buying something nice) or a physical action (taking a week off). Either way, find a way to pat yourself on the ass for a job well done.

However, it's not all moonbeams and unicorn juices; if you fail to achieve your goal, set up a nasty punishment that you will have to endure. Personally, I absolutely loathe doing cardio. It disgusts me. My body actually rejects cardio faster than a hot blonde rejects a hobo. So when I fail to achieve a set goal, my standard self-punishment is a 45 minute treadmill run.

Just the thought of spending close to an hour of my life running like a tool in the exact same spot makes me want to projectile vomit while enduring the visual blasphemy of the Twilight saga. Preferably both at the same time. But it also makes me want to HUSTLE my ass off so that I don't have to go through it.

So find something you hate doing, then set that up as your punishment. Other honorable mentions when it comes to self-punishment are as follows:

- Taking out to dinner someone you cannot stand
- Buying presents for a relative you cannot stand
- Self induced anal probing (unless you like that kind of thing, then it belongs in the reward section)
- Doing the arctic dip/swim
- Let your friends cut your hair (Ladies, I've heard this one is a real motivator)
- Let your friends do your makeup/styling before going out
- No drinking/partying for X number of days

**BONUS – Accountability**

As if four solid steps weren't enough to transform your goals into tangible results, I've got one extra trick up my sleeve. It's a concept that most "life coaches" base their entire business on when helping their clients achieve whatever the hell it is they want to achieve. It's called accountability.

When others know of your goals and get involved by holding you accountable for your actions, a whole bunch of psychological triggers get activated. Below is an example of how I held someone accountable by making their goals public.

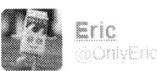 Eric
@OnlyEric

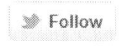 Follow

@FitJerk you're holding me accountable with that retweet. Got to do it now.

← Reply ⤴ Retweet ★ Favorite ⥲ Buffer

6:29 PM - 14 May 12 via Twitter for Android   Embed this Tweet

*The back story: Eric is a dude that generally "knows his stuff" when it comes to training, and after reading my write up on how I overcame low back pain and achieved a National Record deadlift, he said he was inspired to hit up a competition and wanted to achieve a 3x bodyweight pull himself. So, to make sure he wasn't just fluff talking, I retweeted his statement to my 6000+ followers, making it rather public. The screen-shot above was his response to that.*

And it's not just for competitors, this technique can turn the biggest and sloppiest couch-riding dorkwad into a "go get er". The execution is simple: Go up to 5 of your closest friends or family members, hand them a deposit cash amount (the higher the better, such as $50 each) and then tell them your goal, when you plan on reaching that goal and what your planned punishment is should you fail.

If you reach the goal and can prove it to them, they have to give you back that deposit cash amount. If you fail, they get to keep the cash while making sure you don't pussy out on going through the set punishment. As you can probably guess, you'll need some real friends/family members whom you can trust, so don't start handing out cash to mere acquaintances.

If you can follow this four step process (or five step if you're doing the bonus), then there is no way in hell you'll fail. There might be times where you misjudge your deadline so you have to endure your little punishment, but life doesn't stop after that. You just get right back up and keep chugging along. Eventually you'll arrive at your set destination, after which you can give yourself a nice pat on the ass.

Now go get something done.

# Measurements

It should be rather obvious that if you're not tracking your body composition, then you'll never know if you're making progress or not. When I get clients for E-Training, the very first thing I do is tell them to take a before picture and get me their measurements. Until they give me this data, I won't make a plan for them – it really is that important. I've had a few clients which were like, "Oh I'll get you my before picture and measurements next week since [insert lame ass excuse], so can we just get started with the plan?" My usual response to such ridiculousness is, "fuck no."

The ironic thing is that I don't do it to be a "jerk", I do it to showcase the importance of tracking along with dumping a massive amount of accountability onto said client. How fast the plan arrives in their grubby little hands is up to them, and so the next time I'm about to deliver and update to their plan, they know better.

So, what measurements do you need? Well there are 5 sites: Neck, Chest, Waist, Arms and Thighs. Before we dig into the details of where exactly you should measure from, just remember that eliminating additional variables is hella important. That means always use the same tape measure, without flexing, on bare skin and at the same time every week.

You do not want to be tracking the difference in AM and PM times as you usually look "leaner" in the morning due to going 6-8 hours with no food or water. I can't tell you how many times I've had clients measure their bodies at the most random and inconsistent time intervals along with wearing different clothing and then they start freaking out because the progress made wasn't as fast as the week prior.

That type of inconsistent data is absolutely useless. I usually yell at them for not listening and make sure we correct course from there onwards.

Neck – Measure right under the chin or at the thickest point. Men should avoid the Adam's apple and measure right above it.

Chest – Keep it simple, measure right over your nipples and make sure the tape measure stays parallel to the floor. A mirror helps. And if you have nice (man)boobs, it's a fun measurement to do, at least I'd imagine so. And for those with droopy tits, forget the nipples as you're going right across your chest at the arm pit level.

Waist – Some say above the belly button, some say over it but I say right under the belly button. Reason being is that most people who have a belly fat tend to store it close to the groin. Of course, if you rock a true beer belly with a large circumference, then the little details on measuring your gut are negligible. But I like to keep it consistent. So under the ol' button it is.

Arms – You want to measure this ¾ of the way up from the elbow. The reason being is that we want to incorporate the triceps and biceps along with any fat you might be storing. Out of all the measurements, this is the only one I allow to be flexed, especially for guys since the "standard" in arm sizes is measured this way. When you hear about guys that rock 20 inch guns, they measured it flexed. So if you want to do this then go for it, but as always, be consistent.

Thighs – While standing, wrap the tape measure halfway between the knee and hips. To help you track your weekly progress, I've included a chart in Chapter 7. Print that out and throw it up somewhere in your house where you'll see it daily. Better yet, throw it up on a wall where everyone in your house will see it daily. This will do two very important things – First, it will constantly remind you that you should track your progress and second, you and everyone else will see your progress first hand.

Most people think that progress can be visually seen, so why all the measuring? Because minor progress cannot be visually seen!

Try looking at a person with a 35 inch waist versus a person that has a 34 or 34.5 inch waist while having the similar body fat percentages. I guarantee you won't be able to spot the difference, especially if they are wearing clothes. However, when you're taking the effort to better yourself, celebrating every inch matters.

Remember the driving analogy we used earlier? If you happen to embark on a road trip, you only get to see the 50 feet in front of you that your headlights have illuminated - but that's all you need. Feet by feet, you eventually make it to your destination.

So just like a long ass road trip, each inch should be recorded and reflected upon. Otherwise you'll be waiting weeks or even months for noticeable visual differences in your body composition, which will make you cry and quit. The only thing worse than a quitter, is a crying quitter. What a bunch of sorry souls those are. Don't ever cry to quit. Cry to keep going.

## Optional – Body Fat ~~Measurements~~ Guesstimations

If you want to go the extra mile, you may want to invest in a tool that tells you your current bodyfat percentage. Personally, I don't really use this for my clients since calculating the difference in their measurements gives me a rough idea where they're at. Then there's the factor of tool availability – since I train clients from all around the world, a tool someone uses in France will be different than the tool someone uses in Australia and so I cannot assist them with calculations etc. It's too much of a headache to deal with.

However, I do use body fat percentages for my own body. The reason is more public then personal – because when you're this lean and somewhat "popular" on the internet, people tend ask you what your body fat percentage is at. So I like to have an accurate answer. There are a few ways to know your body fat percentage, I'll list them in no particular order below:

Body Fat Calipers – Also known as skin fold calipers. Not only are they relatively inexpensive, but the calipers are still the most accurate tool when you consider "bang of the buck." The problem is that different companies have different formulas. My recommendation is to go for a caliper where the accompanying formula asks for the most number of skin fold sites.

So just as an example, a caliper set that asks for 4 sites is not as accurate as a caliper that asks for 6, 8 or even 12 sites. Don't get too hung up on it though, just buy one and stick with it because as you know all too well by now, consistency is king.

The BodPod – This space age looking thing has recently become popular, probably because it looks like a delicious hard-boiled egg and I want to fondle Scarlett Johansson inside its cozy interior. Unfortunately though, fondling is probably all it's good for since the BodPod rocks an error rate as high as 15%. Which means you have a better chance of guessing your own body weight after night of heavy drinking and staring at the mirror in your green spandex shorts.

James Krieger, who has a masters in Nutrition and in Exercise Science, summarized the BodPod quite effectively by saying, "The Bod Pod does OK when looking at group averages, with some studies showing error rates of around 2%; however, other studies have indicated average error rates of over 5% 1-2. The individual error rate for the Bod Pod can be unacceptably high in some individuals, and the Bod Pod is horrible for tracking change over time. For these reasons I would recommend against using the Bod Pod as a body composition assessment tool. Hydrostatic weighing, despite some of its problems, is much more reliable."

[To read the entire article where he rips the BodPod apart, go here: **http://weightology.net/weightologyweekly/?page_id=175**]

Hydrostatic Weighing – This is when you are (temporarily) drowned to see how much water you are displacing, or in caveman terms, to see how much space your ass takes up.

Then math magicians do a whole bunch of funky shit like calculate your body's density - since fat tends to float and is less denser than muscle, and come up with your body fat percentage. For completeness's sakes, I'll quote my man James Krieger on his thoughts on Hydrostatic Weighing:

"The bottom line is that underwater weighing can give good results when looking at group averages, but not so good results when looking at individuals. The sad thing is that underwater weighing is actually the best method out of the 2-compartment models. Other methods, including the Bod Pod, BIA, and skinfolds, are significantly worse."

[For more on hydrostatic weighing, go here: **http://weightology.net/weightologyweekly/?page_id=162**]

My suggestion is that if you have a facility that does hydrostatic weighing near your area, go do it twice. Once in the beginning, before you start and once again when you are at your goal weight. It's a bitch of a process though, I won't lie. If you are someone who runs out of patience quicker than Gordon Ramsay at dinner service, you might need to bring additional emotional support.

BIA (Bioelectrical Impedance) – This is the method which most of the "high end" weight scales use. The way it works is rather simple; it sends a current through your body and since fat contains very little water compared to muscles, it takes into account your weight and does the magic math required to spit out a body fat percentage. Sounds fancy but my personal recommendation is that you shouldn't even bother - it's useless.

If you happen to step on a BIA scale at some point in your life, don't take the number you see seriously. It's a horrible guess at best. In fact, I have a theory: an experienced coach with a keen eye can look at your regular measurements and predict a more accurate body fat percentage than a BIA scale.

## "Do I Need A Gym Membership?"

N<sub>o.</sub>

But let me tell you, having one sure doesn't hurt! It's completely true that you can get the job done with a pair of resistance bands and bodyweight exercises at home - and if anyone tells you otherwise, punch them directly in the face for lying. But what's not a lie, is that there are some major exercises which you won't be able to perform (such as the deadlift, barbell squat etc.) and therefore your results will come slower.

Why?

Because these are king daddy exercises which engage the largest number of muscle groups, which means they burn the most calories, fire up your metabolism to the max and elicit the biggest release of fat-burning/muscle-building hormones from the body.

Another problem is that you'll be deprived of a very key variable in your training – the load. Unless you are using thick resistance bands and get really creative, it's hard(er) to increase the load of a bodyweight exercise. So if you can live with these two slight drawbacks, then no, you don't need a gym membership, which means you can stop reading this and move on to the *Essential Equipment* section.

If however, you feel that the benefits of having a gym membership is important, and are now considering getting one, let me point you in the right direction so you don't get royally screwed up the behind by those savvy salesmen. Or saleswomen.

On second thought, I don't really mind being screwed by women, it's rather nice.

## FJ's Gym Checklist

**Forget fancy facilities!** You need functionality over aesthetics so don't go for the gym with the biggest number of complicated machines. It might look awe-inspiring, but it's all for show. In fact you should do the opposite - join a gym that has more emphasis on free-weights than machines (if this type of gym happens to be fancy, then that's an exception).

Examples of things to look for inside: Squat Racks, Power Racks, Smith Machine (sounds contradictory but Google it if you don't know what it is), Bench Press Stations (flat, incline and decline), Rowing Station, Pullup Station, A Huge Selection Of Dumbbells (Should at least go up to 8olbs or higher), Ez curl bar with station, Straight bars and finally, a big selection of plates (not just nickels[1-3] and dimes[1-4] lying around).

**No Contracts if possible!** If you cannot avoid this, be sure to check for renewal terms (some companies will auto-renew your membership yearly without telling you) and cancellation of contract fees (which can rage in hundreds of dollars). Bottom line is this: Read the contract before you sign that shit - I cannot stress this enough! And once you are ready to pay, always use a credit card. Never link your bank account directly to their system in any way shape or form.

**Amenities** – If you are signing up for a Premium/Classy looking gym, then make sure they have a steam room/sauna, proper showers and/or a pool. There is no reason to pay a premium if you aren't getting premium features.

**Avoid Planet Fitness...** and other gyms like it. These are the stupid "trendy" gyms where the space is filled with machines, the people are pure hipsters, the dumbbells are lighter than my chestnuts on a wet day, and they look down upon (or even ban) customers who happen to grunt once in a while. What a load of garbage.

If you are paying for a gym to get in a decent workout, make sure it allows you to *really* workout. The gym I go to has big dudes, small dudes, grunting bodybuilders, hot chicks and the fittest moms you'll ever see - and we all manage to workout in harmony. There is no reason other places can't achieve this as well.

**Don't Be Intimidated** if you happen to walk into a gym and everyone looks "advanced". As long as the gym meets our criteria, it's all good. The truth is that people are too busy thinking about themselves which means they don't care as to who you are. Take comfort in that. No one is judging you, because they are too scared to be judged themselves. To be the best, you must ignore the rest.

**Take a test drive.** Most, if not all gyms will let you try out their facility for free and will give you a tour. Free trial times can range from a few days to a few weeks or sometimes a few months if you happen to walk in while they are having some kind of promo. I suggest you bring a notepad when you get the free tour so you can check off what the gym has and doesn't have. *But under no circumstances are you to plunk down your cash before trying out the gym and seeing how it works for you.* If they won't let you take a test drive, then you take your business elsewhere. Remember who is running the show here.

**Don't be swayed by free swag.** A lot of places will offer limited bonuses such as free "consultations" or free detox kits and other nonsense supplements. This is all well and good if you've already *decided* to join the gym but do not let this be a deciding factor in choosing one gym over another. Getting a free shirt or having some dude tape measure your ass for free isn't worth paying more if 2 weeks down the road, you are dissatisfied with the facility.

# Essential Equipment

If you've decided that joining a gym is not an option but you still want the benefits of lifting, then you my friend, will have to invest in your own equipment. This can be quite a blessing since you never have to wait around for people to finish - such as the gutless chumps that are doing bicep curls inside the squat rack (if I catch you doing this, so help me god...)

**The Basics**

**1. A Power Rack:** There is nothing you cannot do with a Power Rack.

Squats? Check.
Bench? Check.
Deadlift? Check.
Rackpull? Check.
Monkey Sex? Check.

There are a million different types, so just look for the following basic features and you should be good to go: Full rack (not a half power rack), adjustable pins, adjustable J-Hooks, attached pullup/chinup bar at the top, slots for your weight plates. Optional features include: Olympic platform, dynamic band pegs, adjustable dip attachments. Expect to spend anywhere from $500 - $2000 on a your rack (uh, not *that* kind of rack).

I will say that once you buy yourself a really good powerack, you probably won't need much else. If you're feeling super creative, find a local welder and ask him to make you one – it may or may not work out cheaper than actually buying one. Good welders only need to look at the picture in order to create something almost as similar and just as functional.

**2. Standard Olympic Barbell:** Depending on the deal you get on the power rack, a bar may or may not come with it. While buying a bar isn't a complicated process, be sure to check how much load it can handle before you buy it. The cheap ones won't be able to hand more than 400lbs – which may seem like a lot until you want to do rack pulls or squat lockouts and realize that you need 500lbs. So just get one with a decently high load threshold. **Buy nice, so you don't gotta buy twice!**

**3. Standard Olympic Weights:** Again, a pretty simple procedure. I suggest buying plates that have handles and/or grips. An every better option would be to buy Olympic bumper plates so you can drop the load when needed. This is huge for safety – there have been plenty of times where I couldn't manage to lift the weights I thought I could, and as such all I had to do was dump it. Bumper plates for the win.

**4. Foam Roller or The Stick:** These are must-have items. You can have both or just stick to one, it doesn't matter. You'll be doing myofascial release on a daily basis – no exceptions. My review for the stick can be found on **http://fitjerk.com/the-stick-review/**

**5. Chalk:** If you have no grip, you have no lift. If you use dorky gloves, you hands will stink like doo-doo. Chalk is the cheapest and most used piece of "equipment" I own. Until it runs out of course, then I have to send out my ~~slave~~ assistant to buy more. You're looking for Magnesium Carbonate – also known as gymnastics chalk or rock climbing chalk. Get some. If your gym doesn't allow it, sneak it in anyway and don't make a mess. If they keep bitching, apologize, then keep lifting.

## Optional Shit You Might Like

**1. Resistance Bands:** These come in handy when you're traveling. They are the best ones I've ever used and are quite convenient to carry.

They have a different strength curve than traditional weights, so they can help by adding new stimulus to your training. You can also replace pretty much any gym exercise with bands.

**2. Fat Gripz:** You can read my entire review on them here: **http://fitjerk.com/fatgripz-review/**. Basically, they attach onto a bar and make them "fatter". A fatter bar requires greater grip strength and that's exactly what this improves. I love these things as they are not only cost effective, but bulletproof. I've made like Chris Brown on 'em and given these things a serious beating - and they still look as good as new. Unlike Chris Brown though, I don't hit women... except maybe on the ass for good behavior. Or sometimes bad behavior.

**3. Manta Ray:** It attaches on to a bar and makes squatting 10x more comfortable and more stable, which results in you lifting more weight. For 95% of you, this thing will probably be a god send. While that sounds exciting, I do not want you to use the Manta Ray initially. It will become a crutch. And not just any crutch – you will end up dependent on it like a broke loser on welfare. You need to learn to squat with a bar on your back. Yes, it's initially uncomfortable. Yes, you might cry.

But give it about 2-4 weeks and the pain will be a non issue. Then introduce the Manta Ray for the occasional max squat session and watch your numbers rise faster than an Apple stock. *(Note: If you're reading this 40 years from now and Apple is in the shitter, know that there was once a time when over-priced, under powered computers and gadgets which relied on bloatware software were a 'hip' thing to purchase)*

My Manta Ray review can be found here: **http://fitjerk.com/product-review-manta-ray-by-advanced-fitness-inc/**

# Chapter 1 References

1-1: Less body fat improves physical and physiological performance in army soldiers.

1-2: Effect of race and musculoskeletal development on the accuracy of air plethysmography.

1-3: A "nickel" is the slang term for a 5lbs plate

1-4: A "dime" is the slang term for a 10lbs plate

1-5: If you have the printed version of the book, use this link: http://www.fitjerk.com/bodylastics

# Chapter 2: What You <u>Should</u> Want In Your Mouth (Nutrition)

# What Are Macronutrients?

The standard definition states that "macronutrients are nutrients that are needed by the body in large quantities". Some people tend to get confused when "macro" and "large quantities" are used in the same sentence, but what they are confusing it with is micronutrients - which are needed by your body in small amounts. So remember, macro = more, micro = less.

So what exactly are these nutrients that we need to consume in large quantities? There are only three: Protein, Carbohydrates (Carbs) & Fats. Be sure to remember these, as well as the order they are written in.

## Protein

Also known as polypeptides; they are found in the cells of all living things and are essential to health. Most of the protein that is in our bodies is made up of about 20 different amino acids. This list of 20 is divided into two groups: Essential Amino Acids and Nonessential Amino Acids.

Essential amino acids must be taken in through diet because the body cannot synthesis them on its own. This is one of the major reasons I don't recommend vegetarianism; plants and vegetables are lacking essential amino's while meat is a complete source of protein. So why the hell wouldn't you eat both? In fact, "vegetarian" was the term our ancient ancestors used to describe the village idiot who couldn't hunt or fish. True story.

While on one hand we have Essential amino acids, on the other we have Nonessential amino acids. I personally hate these terms because it makes it seem that one group is more important than the other, which is definitely not the case.

The only reason the second group is called "non-essential" is because the body can synthesis these amino acids on its own. All 20 amino acids are important for optimal health, just remember that.

**Carbohydrates (Carbs)**

Where the hell do I even begin with carbs? It's one of the most feared macronutrients, to the point where it seems like some people have a phobia of it (Carbophobia?)

Whatever, I'm here to say that you don't need to fear carbs like those panzies. What you do need to do, is figure out which types of carbs to eat, when to eat them and in what quantities. Carbohydrates are the body's primary source of fuel - point blank period.

Let me go on a tangent for a second and take this fuel analogy a bit further - assume you have a car with a tank that can hold 50 gallons of fuel. What happens when you try and pour in more than 50 gallons? Well, either the gas pump will start to "click" or you'll experience the benefits of having an underwear full of gasoline.

Unfortunately (or fortunately) our bodies handle over-fueling a bit differently. It just stores the extra fuel for later use (in the form of fat). Looking at the general population, if the human body's primary reaction was to induce huge diarehheatic shits every time a person "over-fueled" themselves, we wouldn't have an obesity problem.

This book would instead be called Flawless Fitness 2: How to figure out your daily food requirements so you don't randomly crap your pants. If only. Ok enough talking about poop, let's get back on point. It's time to talk about the types of carbohydrates that we need to be concerned with: Low Glycemic/High Glycemic and New Age/Old Age.

## Low Glycemic/High Glycemic Carbohydrates

The Glycemic index, or GI, ranks carbohydrates according to their effect on our blood glucose levels. Foods that are low GI (such as oatmeal, brown rice, whole wheat etc.) cause low fluctuations in our blood glucose and insulin and foods that are high GI (sugar, fructose, white rice etc.) obviously do the opposite. It's those insulin levels which we are really concerned with, especially for fat loss. More on that later.

## New Age/Old Age Carbs

New age carbs refers to foods that we have been consuming for the past few thousand years such as rice, wheat, grains etc. Old age carbs are foods that our species have been consuming since we were cavemen... you know, a time where I could just club dumbasses over the head willingly without getting my ass "sued" and all that bullshit? Those were the good ol' days. Anyways, for more on this particular topic read "Paleo Or Mayo?" in Chapter 3.

## Fats

Alright, so what the hell is fat? Is it the bumpy cellulite you see on the overweight woman at the beach who can't pick her correct thong size? Is it the white stuff surrounding your piece of delicious steak? Or is it the liquid you use to cook your food with? The answer is obviously, "all of the above". I figured I'd start off easy before we go in, ahem, deep and heavy.

The actual scientific term for fat is **lipids,** as it's insoluble in water. Think of lips, then think of lids. Lipids, easy. There are 3 types of lipids that you need to know about for the first 10 seconds... after which I will strip things down butt naked, and you'll only need to know about one.

**The 3 Types Of Lipids:**
**Triglycerides**
**Phospholipids**
**Sterols**

The one were concerned with are the triglycerides because they represent 95% of the fat we consume. Your body happens to store fat in the form of triglycerides as well. The saying "you are what you eat," definitely applies here.

First, let's break down that long ass name; this will help you remember it better. Scientific names are usually logical so once you understand the logic, it will forever click in your brain (unless you're a complete bafoon, then there is no hope).

The word begins with the letters "tri" meaning 3 (duh). This number represents the number of fatty acids, while the term "glyceride" refers to the 3 carbon atom backbone to which the fatty acids are attached to. Below is a little illustration that will help you visualize nature's very own threesome.

```
|G|====[Fatty Acid 1]==========
|L|
|Y|
|C|====[Fatty Acid 2]====
|E|
|R|
|O|
|L|====[Fatty Acid 3]=======
```

With me so far? Cool. Next thing you need to know is that the length of the fatty acid molecule isn't always the same... just as how the length of a man's "manhood" isn't always the same. This is being accurately represented by the illustration above; fatty acid 1 is definitely way more excited to be attached to glycerol than fatty acid 2. Fatty acid 3 on the other hand, is quite content with being average.

However, unlike humans, the chain length of triglycerides are divided into three varieties. We have Short-Chain Fatty Acids, Medium-Chain Fatty Acids and Long-Chain Fatty Acids.

- **Short Chain** represents a fatty acid length of 6 carbon atoms or less
- **Medium Chain** represents a fatty acid length of 6-12 carbon atoms
- **Long Chain** represents a fatty acid length of 14 or more carbon atoms

Why are chain lengths important? Because it will determine the speed and method of digestion as well as the function of the fat you eat. More on which fats to eat will be discussed later.

**Levels Of Saturation**

Ok so we know that a triglyceride is a type of lipid and comes in three varieties: short chain, medium chain and long chain. But annoyingly, triglycerides can also be categorized by the type of carbon atom bonds found inside the fatty acid. If the carbon atoms in a fatty acid is bonded together by single bonds only, we call that **saturated fat**. "What exactly is it saturated by", you ask? Hydrogen!

Every carbon atom in that chain has 2 hydrogen atoms attached to it, for company. Some would say I'm saturated by women. If I was reborn as a fatty acid, you can bet I'd be saturated and "very bad" for your health. As you can see in the diagram below, saturated fat forms a very neat and clean looking molecule... this means that a bunch of them could be packed tightly together resulting in solids at room temperature. Think butter and lard. But it's not always a solid, there are a few exceptions such as coconut oil and palm kernel oil.

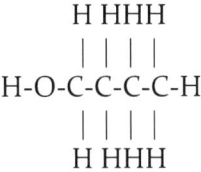

```
  H HHH
  | | | |
H-O-C-C-C-C-H
  | | | |
  H HHH
```

However, if the fatty acid chain has two carbon atoms that are attached together by a DOUBLE BOND, it's called **mono-unsaturated fat**. Mono refers to the number of double bonds in the entire chain (one) and it's unsaturated because at the carbon double bond location, it's not pimping as many hydrogen atoms as saturated fat. Still with me? Good.

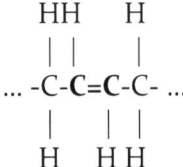

```
  HH    H
  | |   |
... -C-C=C-C- ...
  |   | |
  H   H H
```

The diagram above represents the double-bond section of this particular fatty acid molecule. The shape of a monounsaturated molecule isn't as neat as saturated fat. If you were playing Tetris, this molecule would be like the annoying "Z" block that's a pain in the ass to slot away neatly. And as such, at room temperature, it's found in the form of liquids (olive oil, canola oil etc.)

And finally we have a third type of triglyceride called **poly-unsaturated fat**. "Poly" because it's got more than one double bond, and "unsaturated" because just like monounsaturated fat, it can't pimp too many hydrogen atoms at its double bond locations (See diagram on next page). Again, just like with monounsaturated fat this molecule has a messy shape, and therefore comes in the form of liquids. Alpha Linoleic acid is one example, while other oils include cottonseed, corn and safflower.

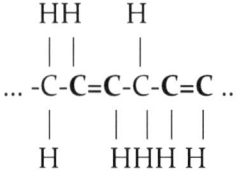

## Piecing The Fatness Together

The final thing you need to know is that foods rarely contain *one* type of triglyceride. They all contain a mix of everything you've read above. For example, butter is 65% saturated fat, 31% monounsaturated fat and 4% polyunsaturated fat. But because the majority of its construction at a molecular level is saturated, it stays solid at room temperature. And gets even more solid when you put it in the fridge, at which point it won't spread nicely on your toast.

Don't holes in your toast totally piss you off? Yeah, me too.

On the flipside we have olive oil which contains 14% saturated fat, 74% monounsaturated fat and 10% polyunsaturated fat which is why it's a liquid. Also, for future reference I'll be using acronyms when talking about the different type of triglycerides to make things easier. They are listed below... get to know them as well as, if not better than your spouse. If you're lonely and have no spouse, then get to know them better than your right hand.

**SFA** = Saturated Fatty Acid
**MUFA** = Monounsaturated Fatty Acid
**PUFA** = (...take a wild guess; consider it a pop quiz)

So why did I bother with such an exhaustive overview on fat? Because the biggest fear most people have is that if you *eat* fat, you'll *get* fat. While this statement has some validity to it (especially when your calories rack up), it is only partially true since the *quality of food matters*. So don't be like most people, and realize that all calories are *not* equal[2-4]!

What you need to be concerned with is the types of dietary fats you consume, and that's about it. There are good fats and bad fats. Good fats such as Omega-3/6/9 fatty acids, polyunsaturated and monounsaturated fats are more beneficial than saturated and trans fats.

Having said that, don't think that I'm telling you to completely cut out saturated fats because in moderation it has a specific job to do. Trans fatty acids from natural animal meat is not something you need to get your panties in a bunch about. It's the hydrogenated garbage in things such as potato chips you need to avoid.

Also, good sources of natural saturated fat such as butter, is not a big freakin' deal. Butter tastes awesome, why would you completely avoid it? As long as you remember to count the amount you ate towards your daily macronutrient limits, you'll be just dandy.

Now here's a little trick (other than switching to virgin olive oil for cooking needs), look into consuming fats that are known as medium-chain-triglycerides (MCT's). The beauty of MCT's is that in about a few hours after ingestion, they are readily available to the tissues in your body (such as muscles) as fuel. Also, from what I've experienced and read, they are hardly ever *stored* as fat in your body!

MCT's also spare protein, which means when you are cutting down on carbs, your body won't be sexually eyeing your muscles as a fuel source. This is very crucial to our goals because remember - we want to lose fat while minimizing muscle loss. Google MCT oils if you want to try some.

# FJ's Take On Dairy

$A$h yes the huge controversy that is dairy. Since there are so many people with strong opinions on dairy... I'm going to give you my personal take on this overblown shit-show and how I manage to deal with it. We in North America consume more dairy products than anybody else in the world! We have so much that in the past, our governments have spent millions of dollars trying to store the surplus of milk (I wouldn't be surprised if this is going on right now).

Ever seen those ads that promote milk? Of course you have, we all get bombarded with them at random times during the year. It might seem odd but those ads aren't just meant to increase sales, they are used to reduce the surplus they've amassed. It is often said that North America alone produces enough food to feed the entire world... whether that statement is true or not isn't the point.

The point is that we have way too much food, therefore its availability is high and price is low. But with high quantity also comes a loss in quality, which is why the dairy products of today are "fortified" with growth  hormones, vitamins, minerals and whatever else is lacking inside in order to make it equal to its organic counterpart.

The original (and often convincing) argument used to be that since most animals in nature don't consume milk from other species, then it is logical to assume that humans should also avoid drinking milk from cows. When you look at the data, it further drives the point home (65-70% of adults are lactose intolerant). Below is a chart which represents the Ethnicity group along with their % lactose intolerance.

| Ethnicity/Geo Region | % Lactose Intolerance | Ethnicity/Geo Region | % Lactose Intolerance |
|---|---|---|---|
| 1. East Asian | 90-100 | 10. Latino / Hispanic | 51 |
| 2. Indigenous | 80-100 | 11. Indian (North) | 30 |
| 3. Central Asian | 80 | 12. Anglo (NA) | 21 |
| 4. African American | 75 | 13. Italian (Italy) | 20-70 |
| 5. African (African) | 70-90 | 14. French (North) | 17 |
| 6. Indian (South) | 70 | 15. Finnish | 17 |
| 7. French (south) | 65 | 16. Austrian | 15-20 |
| 8. Jewish | 60-80 | 17. German | 15 |
| 9. Balkans Region | 55 | 18. British (UK) | 5-15 |

But then, even though we have all this data[2-1] the simple fact of the matter remains -humans have been consuming milk and dairy products for a long ass time, and we've been doing just fine. Alan Aragon, a solid nutritionist whom I respect, puts the whole dairy hoopla to rest by saying,

*"Are you kidding me? So who gets to decide which parts of the cow we should consume? Let me get this straight–we can eat the cow's muscles, but not the milk that laid the foundation for the growth of those same muscles? Huh? The logic is just too rock-solid for me."*

**The Bottom Line**

At the end of the day, the truth is that you are most likely intolerant to milk and/or dairy products to some degree. To you, milk is either the catalyst to huge diuretic shits, something that causes mild discomfort, or a liquid that does nothing but good to your body without ill consequences.

Only you know where your relationship with dairy products lies. But regardless of how your body reacts to it, one thing is for certain - the benefits of dairy far outweigh its faults...

- Whey protein is quick absorbing and a staple for anyone looking to get lean.
- Ice cream is straight up, fucking delicious.
- Pizza would be nothing without the different types of cheeses melted on top.
- Chocolate milk... well it's the same color as me, so it's awesome by default.
- Regular milk is full of goodness and breakfast cereals would be lonely without it.
- Coffee by itself is ok, but orally orgasmic the moment you add cream.
- Whip cream can be eaten off sensual body parts.

I think you get my point; a life sans dairy products is rather empty and meaningless... unless of course, you're deathly allergic to it. But even then, think about it for a second; you can die happy eating ice cream or attempt to kill yourself with a ShakeWeight™ while choking down bland "healthy" egg whites. I don't know, but I think the former is a much more exciting option if you feel like becoming part of history, but I'll let you decide*.

Ok let's get back on track, so what should you do at this point? You being a person that is looking to get lean and for whatever reason, live as long as you possibly can. Should you avoid dairy? Or should you just say, "screw it, I love my cows!" and keep on enjoying it? The answer actually lies somewhere in the middle. While Aragon's statement is hilariously true, don't forget, so is the data.

I find that if I eat dairy for too long without taking a break from it, things start to get funky on the insides. My solution is a quarterly break from the goodness that comes out of the cow's titties.

Depending on how sensitive you are to it, your break cycle may vary. I started by taking two weeks off dairy and noticed that I had less mucus buildup along with a less sensitive nose to summer allergies. Your results and experiences will vary, but you should notice a difference.

From there, start introducing dairy products into your meal plan and notice when the "ill effects" start to appear once again. As soon as they do, go off dairy for a week. If it took a month, then you know that once a month you need to do a mini dairy detox. If it took a week, you might need to alternate weeks. But this can get tedious, so my solution for these folks is to forget the dairy detox cycle and just consume less and/or supplement with digestive enzymes.

Having said all of that, if by doing a two week dairy detox didn't produce a noticeable difference in your energy, mood, irritability etc., then you should be glad, because you're probably not allergic and have no intolerances[2-2] to dairy products. But if you're such a person, then you already knew that.

*Just to be clear, killing yourself is not an option. Suicide is the loser's way out.*

# Highly Fucked Corny Syrup (HFCS)

When it comes to HFCS (ok, it actually stands for *high fructose corn syrup*), you might have heard about how it's all "bad", "poisonous" and most likely conjured in the evil depths of a witch's basement where she also keeps naughty bondage gear. Not so. HFCS is simply made up of glucose and fructose. You can tell how much of each is within the syrup, defined by the number.

So if you see HFCS-55, it is comprised of 55% fructose and the rest is glucose. The number always represents how much fructose it contains so if you want to find its glucose amount, use simple mathematical elimination. If you can't, go back to grade 5.

I'd say the bigger problem is the media - which has scared the shit out of the general population by making blanket statements such as, "consuming HFCS makes you fat, and studies[2-6] prove it!" This "study" which many seem to point at was completely useless due to two reasons:

First, because it was done on rats and not humans. Now usually, doing studies on rats isn't a bad thing, as their metabolism is similar to ours, but it has been shown that rats are more sensitive to HFCs[2-7] and their bodies are way more efficient at converting carbohydrate into fat than ours, which already puts them at a slight disadvantage. But a rat's superior carbohydrate converting capability isn't the main reason why I think this study was bullshit. No. The main reason is that the dose of sugar given to the rats was so ridiculous, if you were to convert that amount for average human consumption, it would equal about 3000 calories.

Now understand that an average person eats around 1500-2000 calories a day from regular food, so they're telling us that eating 3000 calories a day in pure sugar will make a person fat? Really? No fucking way!

Please dear scientists, why don't you carry out further studies that will reveal conclusions so obvious, that a person high on acid wouldn't have an issue predicting.

And there were other problems with it as well, but at this point it doesn't matter. They should've just spent the research money at a local strip joint and fed the nice, hard-working ladies some sugar instead. It would've been a more worthwhile investment, if you ask me.

So what's my stance on HFCS? Simple -- avoid when possible. It'll surprise you to know that my major concern isn't the molecular make up High Fructose Corn Syrup, it's actually corn itself. You see, most corn that you can buy today - 90% of it - is genetically modified (GMO) and comes from farms that are under the tight vice grip of a chemical giant known as Monsanto. If you know not the evil that is Monsanto, nor have you ever watched the documentary Food Inc., then let me bring your dated ass up to speed.

Sometime around the 1980's the American government decided that it'll approve the ability for anyone to patent life (which is absurd), and so Monsanto came up with a soybean seed which contained its own patented gene. Why was this necessary when we already have a natural alternative? Well since Monsanto's a chemical company, they had a product known as Round Up, which was basically a pesticide. Now usually, if you sprayed Round Up on anything (including natural seeds) it would destroy them completely. You wouldn't be wrong in saying that Round Up was a shotgun approach to pest control. However, there was one type of seed it didn't kill – Monsanto's own patented soybean seed. How fucking convenient is that?

In theory, having a seed which can resist a pesticide that has the ability to destroy everything in its path is a match made in heaven - because you can plant as much as you want without having to worry about potential losses.

And so, armed with the perfect marketing angle, Monsanto went around to farmers by saying their miracle duo will kill pests, improve profitability, reduce work time and slash overall costs associated with the traditional method of growing corn – which involves saving their own seeds and planting it again the following season. Sounds all well and good, but the truth of the matter is that Monsanto is comprised of ruthless assholes that managed to forcefully bend over every farmer and screwed em' hard. Here's how...

First of all, once you buy the Round Up ready soybean seeds, you will have to keep buying seeds for the rest of eternity due to contractual obligations. The old, tried and true method of saving your own seed - which has been used for over 10,000 years - wasn't allowed. If you tried to save your own seed, and Monsanto found out, they'd sue the ever loving shit out of you since they own the patent to their seed. So if you're planting it, you gotta play by *their* rules.

But what if you hold up the middle finger and decide not to farm the Monsanto way? You're still at risk. Say a farm right next to yours is using Round Up and the Round Up ready soybean seed. If pollen from their farm blows over to yours, or if there is some form of contamination due to natural causes, *you* are still held accountable.

Why?

Because technically, you now have Monsanto's intellectual property on your land. They don't care how it got there, just the fact that it's there is enough to get your ass sued. This, along with other ruthless tactics is how Monsanto controls over 90% of the corn production - and I haven't even gotten to the worst bit yet...

While it's bad enough that people who produce our food are being screwed and controlled by Monsanto, the product that comes out of their land is of inferior quality.

There was a study[2-8] done recently where rats were fed maize grown from Round Up ready seeds, and here's what they found:

*"In a study published in "Food and Chemical Toxicology", researchers led by Professor Gilles-Eric Seralini from CRIIGEN have found that rats fed on a diet containing NK603 Roundup tolerant GM maize or given water containing Roundup, at levels permitted in drinking water and GM crops in the US, developed cancers faster and died earlier than rats fed on a standard diet. They suffered breast cancer and severe liver and kidney damage."*

Now earlier I mentioned how using rats for the HFCS study wasn't a great idea, but there *is* a very good reason why these rodents are used in toxicology studies – rats don't live too long, and fuck like crazy. This means you can study the long term effects of a chemical by observing the changes in a rat's health over a majority of its lifetime, along with any birth defects in its future generations.

The Round Up seed has been around for slightly longer than a decade, so understanding its long term effects on humans would require studies that last something like 50 years. No one has the time or patience for that shit, therefore rats are used instead.

So basically, if a rat ingests a certain substance and starts to develop cancer and/or other very large tumors within a few months, it's a pretty good indication that years down the line, you'll be just as screwed as our trusty rodent. This was definitely the case with the CRIIGEN study.

I don't know about you, but at this point, organic food is looking more appealing than morning sex on a tropical beach.

So let's wrap up this whole corn debacle. I realize that at this point, it may seem like I'm going back and forth like an Asian ping-pong match. On one hand, I'm saying that HFCS is actually not that bad in structure and function, which is true. But on the other hand, the raw ingredient from where it comes from is so fucked beyond belief that it is quite possibly dangerous to your health, which is also true.

So what should you, the average consumer, do?

As I sated earlier, avoid HFCS as much as possible. When it comes to grocery shopping, opt for organic options. Remember, it's not corn syrup that is making people fat - the real reasons behind people becoming horizontally challenged is due to the general rise in caloric intake, period[2-8,9]. People are, on average eating more and moving less. Yes, the quality of food in general has dropped, but not if you know where to look.

# Trendy Foods Are Bullshit!

"Trendy foods" is the new term I use to describe the latest food products that are created or devised by men in lab coats and nerdy glasses in an attempt to perfect mother nature (GMO's would fit this category). The worst part is that these fake ass products are preached by the "trendy trainers" to their clients. More like trendy douchepuppets! Two immediate and well-known examples that come to mind are: egg substitutes and margarine.

Let me give you something to think about... the ingredients in butter are: *Cream & Salt*. The ingredients in margarine: *Liquid Canola Oil, Water, Partially Hydrogenated Soybean Oil, Plant Stanol Esters, Salt, Emulsifiers, (Vegetable Mono/Diglycerides, Soy Lecithin), Hydrogenated Soybean Oil, Potassium Sorbate, Citric Acid and Calcium Disodium EDTA to Preserve Freshness, Artificial Flavor, DL-alpha-Tocopheryl Acetate, Vitamin A Palmitate, Color.*

Do you really think that it is more beneficial to eat margarine instead of butter? You're a moron if you do.

The message here is simple: **stop ingesting these stank-ass fake foods and stick to the original stuff!** Egg whites and Egg substitutes are bullshit. The amount of nutrition found whole eggs is absolutely awesome. Don't worry about the extra cholesterol, its good cholesterol.

Unless you are regularly eating something like 15 eggs a day, it won't have any negative effects on you. I myself eat 6 eggs a day... and do I look like I have a fucking cholesterol problem?

One of the greatest strength coaches of all time, Charles Poliquin, says that "egg whites are for dorks" and Alan Aragon (nutrition M.D) says "mother nature cringes every time an egg yolk hits the waste basket".

I strongly agree with both these individuals, and you should too. It is so much easier to enjoy the natural foods in conservative quantities than lathering on the fake shit and assuming there will be no consequences in the future.

## List Of Real Foods & Their Fake Counterparts To Avoid

| | |
|---|---|
| Eggs | Egg Whites/Substitutes |
| Milk | Powdered Nonsense |
| Cream | Non-Dairy Creamer |
| Cheese | Processed Plastic |
| Bacon | Turkey Bacon |
| Butter | Margarine |
| Lean Cut Of Beef | Soy Burger |
| Sugar | Aspartame |
| Water | Vitamin Water® |

# The Ultimate Food Guide

Almonds
Apples
Asparagus
Artichokes
Bananas
Bread (brown, rye, whole wheat)
Broccoli or Broccoli Sprouts
Beans
Beets
Beef (lean cuts)
Buffalo
Blueberries
Bran
Brussels Sprouts
Celery
Cabbage
Cantaloupe
Carrots
Cauliflower
Cereal (Whole grain like Raisin Bran)
Citrus fruits
Citrus Juices (Not concentrate)
Cranberry Juice
Cherries
Chicken (Skinless white meat)
Coffee, black
Corn
Cucumbers
Cottage Cheese (Low fat)
Deer Meat
Eggs or Egg whites
Eggplant
Fish, (Cold water salmon, sardines)
Graham Crackers
Garlic (Fresh)

Grape Juice
Kale
Kiwi fruit
Lettuce (romaine)
Lima Beans
Mangoes
Milk (1% or 2%)
Mushrooms
Melons
Nectarines
Oatmeal
Olive Oil
Onions
Ostrich
Oysters
Portobello
Papayas
Peas
Peppers
Prunes
Pancakes (buckwheat)
Pasta with vegetables
Peaches
Peanut Butter (organic)
Pears
Plums
Rice (Brown)
Raisins
Raspberries
Ricotta Cheese
Salsa
Spinach
Sweet Potatoes
Shellfish
Soymilk
Strawberries
String Beans

Sunflower Seeds
Tea (Green or Black)
Tofu
Tomato (sauces or products)
Tuna
Turkey Breast
Vegetable Juice
Veggie Burgers
Walnuts
Watermelon
Wine (RED)
WATER
Yogurt (frozen, non-fat)
Zucchini
**Beef (sirloin)**
**Beer**
**Butter**
**Canadian Bacon**
**Cheese**
**Chili**
**Chinese food**
**Crackers**
**Cream cheese**
**Granola**
**Ham**
**Honey**
**Lettuce (Iceberg)**

What I've just given you, is a fool-proof grocery list. If anything and everything you ever buy comes from the following list, you can be pretty sure that you are eating "healthy". Of course, just because it's healthy does not mean I'm giving you outright permission to disregard quantity, but we'll get to that later.

Now I know most of these seem like ingredients, and obviously some can be eaten by themselves while others can be used to make delicious meals.

Just remember, be creative, and have fun with it (that's important!) Also, please note the foods at the end of the list which are in **bold** lettering. These are foods that must be eaten in moderation, otherwise a virtual replica of my hand will materialize out of these pages and smack you in the head, just like those v8 commercials.

## Dealing with Real Life

Ok, so I have shown you what to eat, but not exactly *how* to eat it (we will get to that in a minute). But let's face it, we live in a world full of uncertainty. As much as I would like you to eat properly 7 days a week, 365 days a year, it is probably not going to happen. You have friends, family and a social life. So how do you deal with the outside pressures of unhealthy foods and drinks?

Well I am glad you asked because that is exactly the question we are going to tackle. If you recall earlier I told you to fill your house with healthy foods and leave no bad choice available – and you *must* practice this... but out of the 7 days in a week, pick one day where you will spoil yourself a little bit. (Don't you dare get carried away with this and have fast-food for breakfast, lunch and dinner. I will E-Smack you - it's a free feature included without your consent)

But just slightly spoiling yourself is cool. Maybe you can have that favorite brownie dessert after you cook yourself a healthy dinner, or maybe you can go out for a beer and some wings with the boys for that big game. This one day will fulfill your crazy cravings and can also be used as a little reward for your hard work and diligence. Go ahead, you deserve it!

Personally, I find that having one 'spoil' day also acts as a great motivator and has me feeling much happier. The funny thing is, since I have formed a habit of eating well I physically cannot eat the bad foods without feeling dull. I tried this out. One day, I *forced* myself to have a burger (from a certain fast food place that I won't mention) for breakfast and lunch. After I ate it I felt weak, miserable and wanted to projectile vomit over the counter.

It just goes to show that your body *can* get used to good foods, you just have to give it some time. (And maybe some love, if needed)

## Intelligent Calorie Partitioning

While having a "spoil day" will work for the average individual, it will really mess with your overall results if you are looking to get ultra lean. The more dramatic the results you want, the tighter control you need to have about what goes in your mouth. So what to do if there is a huge family turkey dinner coming up tomorrow night? Panic? Give up? Not a chance!

Let's assume that you've calculated your daily macro ratios to be (200/100/35) protein, carbs and fat respectively. It's safe to say that almost all family dinners can end up being extremely carb heavy. So all you have to do is take in nothing but protein (which by the way is very satiating so you won't feel too hungry) during the first half of your day.

To put it into perspective, a hundred grams of protein is about three and a half chicken breasts (depending on where you get your chicken from.) By the time you go to this family feast, you'll have an extremely wide margin to meet the rest of your daily caloric requirements.

What's more, if you ate fat free chicken breasts then you have 100g protein, 100g carbs and 35g of fat to play around with. That's 845 calories, which I should say is a hefty amount of food. At this point you don't even have to bother counting, just let loose and eat anything you want.

Chances are, you'll probably get very close to your calculated numbers. Sacrificing carbs in the AM so that you can pig out in the PM is one of the easiest tricks you can pull off. Use it wisely, as it will come in handy on plenty of occasions.

You may also do this if you are planning on going drinking at night. Alcohol is more calorie dense that either protein or carbohydrates so be aware of that. If you plan on getting hammered, leave a slightly bigger window in terms of your macro ratios.

Also, I'd recommend that you stay away from bitch drinks (sugary cocktails.) It's a much better idea (not to mention, way more fun) to do straight shots. I mean if you're gona party, then party hard otherwise what's the fucking point?

TIP:
Here is an interesting fact for all the women out there. Ever since I started eating well, my skin has never felt better. I basically never get pimples and people ask me how I have such great skin. Trust me, no cream out there will make your skin feel this good and radiant! How's that for a positive side effect?!

# The Cons Of Traditional Dieting

Out of all the fitness lingo that is floating around out there, the word "diet" pisses me off the most. Mediterranean Diet, South Beach Diet, Atkins Diet... it seems that anything with the word "diet" at the end of it will sell. It's all horseshit, and I'll tell you why; because the word diet implies a short-term solution. It's also got the word "die" in there which I find highly fitting. Everyone wants to diet, but the harsh reality is that if you want long term success (as in, *keep* an amazing body for life) then you're going to have to incur an eating lifestyle.

You know that Mediterranean Diet? Well to the Mediterranean folks, it's not a damn *diet*... it's a way of life. That marketed diet program is modeled on the way they've been eating for god knows how long, but the program sells because data shows that the Mediterranean population has an above-average lifespan. So the mis-informed consumer makes the logical connection, and thinks they will live just as long if they eat like the Mediterraneans for a few weeks. Hah!

Want to know the absolute worst thing about these mainstream Hollywood-endorsed diets? People rebound off them harder than a meth addict. Why? Because no one knows how long a diet should last. The dieters following the laid out protocols are looking for an ending date - a period where they can let out a sigh of relief, go back to their old miserable ways and assume that everything will be sunshine and rainbows.

Doesn't work like that. Looking good does not have an end date, so please drop this belief immediately. Focus on building a *habit* and you will never have to worry about losing your god like figure ever again.

## The One Exception

While adopting a proper eating habit is *the* way to go, there *is* a time where dieting can be a useful tool. This means you'll follow a strict eating guideline for a set period of time with the aim of achieving accelerated results, then you will go back to your normal eating habits which were great to being with. This type of periodic dieting has a much better name: Carb Cycling - it's a technique which we will discuss in detail in Chapter 3.

For now, I want you to re-read what I wrote above. Actually I've re-pasted it for your convenience: *"follow a strict eating guideline for a set period of time with the aim of achieving accelerated results, then you will go back to your normal eating habits which were great to being with"*.

Can you guess what I'm getting at? Carb Cycling is a technique that is *only* to be used by those who have proper eating habits in place to begin with. Don't think you can just jump right into this technique with body fat levels of 30%, or something equally high, because you will suffer. And more importantly, do more harm than good.

With that said, let's talk about the benefits of carb cycling...

# Reasons Why Carb Cycling Rocks!

Since this technique isn't a long-term sustainable solution, you'll have to determine the frequency which suits you best. I'll give you some pointers later on when we actually discuss *how* to carb cycle. Personally, I carb-cycle about 2-3 times per year and here's why:

1. Allows you to achieve extremely low body fat levels without resorting to expensive drugs and unhealthy dehydration tactics. (Though you *can* use certain supplements and drugs in conjunction with the technique, should you choose. More on that in Chapter 5).

2. Allows you times where you can eat all the junk food you could possibly want! Nope, what you read was not a typo, and nor was it an ingenious attempt to pull a practical joke on your ass (although I've done my fair share of that). If you follow my instructions to a "T" you really *can* go nuts with foods you never would've thought you could eat on a "diet".

3. Builds discipline. This technique is far from easy to pull off, and the first couple times you try it, you won't be able to do it exactly the way it's laid out. No matter, because as you work towards it, you will build discipline and this will affect other areas of your life in a positive way. Think about something significant that you've achieved in life, did you do so in your very first attempt? Highly unlikely. It's the same with Carb Cycling.

4. Gets your body looking fuller and denser than a porn star's erection. Every time I Carb Cycle, my muscle definition is increased and I am clearly more vascular in the gym, without the use of those lame "pump" supplements. And that's about it - I could have come up with other filler reasons but I'm not here to over-hype this technique. Its power is in its effectiveness, as you'll soon see.

# Food Combination Revisited

In my previous book, I talked a bit about food combination theory (FCT) and why I believed it was, for the lack of a better term, fantabulous. This time around though, I'm going to revisit the subject with a bit of a twist. If you're unaware of FCT, the basic concept states that when certain combinations of foods are eaten, they digest with better efficiency and yield a greater energy output than others which can help with weight loss and what have you.

It basically came down to a technique where carbs and protein would not be eaten together, and to hell with fats (poor lipids, no one likes them).

Here's the theory behind it: When you eat protein, the body releases acidic juices to digest it. When you eat carbohydrates, the body releases an alkaline substance - so what happens when acidic and alkaline juices mix? Bam! Instant neutralization. One cancels the other out and the food you ate takes forever to digest resulting in feeling bloated, gaining weight, feeling like shit etc.

Science of course has disproven this, and a study[2-3] done in 2000 showed that it doesn't really matter how you combine the foods, it's not an effective diet strategy. Here were the results they found:

*"There was no significant difference in the amount of weight loss in response to dissociated (6.2 +/- 0.6 kg) or balanced (7.5 +/- 0.4 kg) diets. Furthermore, significant decreases in total body fat and waist-to-hip circumference ratio were seen in both groups, and the magnitude of the changes did not vary as a function of the diet composition.*

*Fasting plasma glucose, insulin, total cholesterol and triacylglycerol concentrations decreased significantly and similarly in patients receiving both diets. Both systolic and diastolic blood pressure values decreased significantly in patients eating balanced diets.*

*The results of this study show that both diets achieved similar weight loss. Total fat weight loss was higher in balanced diets, although differences did not reach statistical significance. Total lean body mass was identically spared in both groups.*

**Conclusion:** *In summary at identical energy intake and similar substrate composition, the dissociated (or 'food combining') diet did not bring any additional loss in weight and body fat."*

Fair enough. And if you really think about it, the fact that FCT was disproven makes sense. Take mother's milk for example – it's composed of all three macronutrients (protein, carbs, fats) and we seem to be able to handle that just fine.

But what studies haven't proved is why you *feel* so god damn fantastic when you do separate carbs from protein. My theory is that while the body has the ability to digest mixed meals, separating them just makes the process more efficient and/or easier for your body. And this isn't just me talking outta my ass, about two-thirds of my previous book holders reported an increase in energy when separating carbs from protein. To the others, I told them they could eat however they wanted.

One final advantage that food combination can have, is that it can be a sneaky way to trick yourself towards a caloric deficit. Think about it, eating the burger without the bun will save you roughly 20g of processed carbohydrates (80 calories). Having wings and ditching the glass of soda will spare you another 100 calories or so. Do this day in and day out, and the little deficits start to add up... or subtract down, whatever. The point is that it will have a favorable result on fat loss, especially when you throw in intense exercise.

So my new opinion on food combination is this: **Try it out.** If it works, then do it as often as possible. If it doesn't work, then mixing and matching is something you can do whenever you feel like it.

Many people talked a lot of nonsense about C.Poliquin's "meat and nut breakfast" that he recommended for his clients. But instead of spending hours arguing with no-life losers on the internet, I pondered over the idea and decided to give it a shot.

The result? An absolute surge in energy levels which has lead me to believe that it's the best way to start your day - bar none (except maybe morning sex, that shit is quite the day starter a well). And it's not only me, my good buddy Jon Goodman[2-5] (a solid trainer in his own right) has also been raving about it publically on twitter and such.

Now think about it – what if I wasted my life arguing with a bunch of wankers who usually have too much time on their hands? I wouldn't have known how awesome the meat and nuts breakfast was, and nor would I have an excuse to devour steak at 9am. In fact, if I based an opinion on pure data alone (of which there is none, as far as I know) I would have ditched the idea, deemed it dumb and would lack a great tool in my toolbox, along with my excuse to eat steak at 9am.

So, back to food combination theory – or more like, food separation theory. While I can't say that my previous customer base models the entire human population accurately, I would bet that FCT (from an energy stand point) works for the majority of people.

**The 7 Day Test**

Here's a simple and easy method to see if food combination is right for you. Again, this won't have an effect on your fat loss goals, but we are after energy enhancements here. Use your smartphone and start a note using some type of note-taking app. You will be using the principals of food combination at every meal and will write down your energy level (on a scale of 1-10) twenty minutes after stuffing your face. So an example log would look like this:

## Monday Feb 16<sup>th</sup> 2043

Meal 1 – 10am (7/10)
Meal 2 – 2pm (8/10)
Meal 3 – 7:30pm (7/10)

As you can see, I've made this example log to be future-proof for the next 31 years. So my offspring can read my masterpiece and hopefully not be walking, talking, physical embarrassments (don't worry, daddy still loves all 14 of you). So back to the log - after seven days you should have a boat load of guesstimated data on how you felt during your little experiment. Now do the exact same experiment without combining your foods.

Keep your rest periods (how long you sleep at night), your energy expenditure (your workouts) and your meal times consistent. The only thing that should change is how you're ingesting your meals. I guarantee that by the end of two weeks, you'll have a clear answer.

### How Long Should I Wait Between My Protein And/Or Carb Meals?

When you separate these macronutrients, a carb meal should be given an hour to digest while a protein meal should be given 2-3 hours. I would also practice alternation so that you can hit your daily macronutrient targets.

And one more thing, vegetables and fruits don't matter. You can eat them with whatever and whenever you like since they have high water content. When the water content is removed though, (such as a baked potato) then it's considered a strict carbohydrate... in which case you only combine it with other carbs.

Simple enough.

# Chapter 2 References

2-1: Lactose Intolerance by Ethnicity and Region

2-2: Ideally, ask your doctor where you can get an intolerance test done. They should test for proteins, gluten and dairy all in one go so you can be sure.

2-3: Similar weight loss with low-energy food combining or balanced diets

2-4: "A calorie is a calorie" violates the second law of thermodynamics

2-5: Visit Jon Goodman's site at www.theptdc.com | Also see his tweet on meat/nut breakfast, and here's him doing some food "separation" of his own. But not because of FCT, but because the poor chap is gluten intolerant. Wrapping in lettuce is a good technique.

2-6: High-fructose corn syrup causes characteristics of obesity in rats: increased body weight, body fat and triglyceride levels

2-7: Comparison of the expression and activity of the lipogenic pathway in human and rat adipose tissue

2-8: http://www.alanaragonblog.com/2010/01/29/the-bitter-truth-about-fructose-alarmism/

2-9: http://www.ers.usda.gov/data-products/food-availability-(per-capita)-data-system.aspx

# Chapter 3: Learn To Walk, Before You Start Running (Fundamentals)

# FJ's Three Golden Laws Of Fat Loss

When you are obsessed with fat loss, you tend do some obsessive things. For me that involved reading countless books and studies, trying a shit load of different supplements and training my ass off. After a while, patterns emerged and it all became very clear. I felt like Neo when he "saw" what the Matrix was for the first time and this allowed me to come up with my 3 golden laws of fat loss.

**These 3 laws of fat loss will not, and cannot be broken. In fact, ANY fat loss system or program that's out there probably follows at least one of these laws (if not all three). If it doesn't, it probably blows chunks and will-not-deliver-results. You can count on it!**

**Fat Loss Law #1: Caloric Restriction**

This law is as simple as it is effective. So many supplement companies are telling you to *consume* this product or that product to achieve rapid fat loss and weight loss. Hmm, let's think about this load of insanity for a second... to *lose* weight and body fat, the food cartels and supplement companies want you to *consume* more of their bullshit.

Can you spot the complete logical disconnect there? And yet, the general population just eats up their lies, then continues to balloon into a shape that has the potential to eclipse my sunshine.

If you want to drop the fat and overall weight, you first need to start *consuming less* than usual. How much less? Well everyone has something called the basal metabolic rate (BMR). This is the amount of calories your body burns off daily to simply keep you alive. For the sake of argument, let's assume that your basal metabolic rate (BMR) is 2000 calories.

So isn't it obvious that if you eat less than your BMR, you will drop weight and if you eat more than your BMR (which a majority of North Americans do) you will gain weight? Duh!

While this type of theoretical caloric math is never 100% accurate, it still gives you a very good idea of what you're doing wrong and why you aren't successful in your venture to look absolutely ripped (Near the end of the book when we put everything together, I'll show you how to increase your accuracy to near perfection). So now the question is: **How exactly do you find your basal metabolic rate?**

Well, you do some math. I know... you vowed never to do math again after you go out of high school, but trust me, it ain't that bad. The hard part is already done for us, we just need to be competent enough to plug some numbers into an equation and enjoy the result it spits out.

It's called the Harris-Benedict Formula...

**For Men**
BMR = 66+(6.23 x weight in lbs) + (12.7 x height in inches) – (6.8 x age in years)

**For Women**
BMR = 655+(4.35 x weight in lbs) + (4.7 x height in inches) – (4.7 x age in years)

**Activity factor**

Sedentary = BMR X 1.2 (little or no exercise, desk job)
Lightly active = BMR X 1.375 (light exercise/sports 1-3 days/wk)
Mod. active = BMR X 1.55 (moderate exercise/sports 3-5 days/wk)
Very active = BMR X 1.725 (hard exercise/sports 6-7 days/wk)
Extremely Active = BMR X 1.9 (daily exercise/sports & physical job or 2X/day training)

As you can see, the formula is pretty straight forward. You throw in the three personal details (weight in lbs, height in inches and age in years) to get your standard BMR. You then take that number and multiply it by your *current* activity factor, not the amount of activity I'll have you do soon.

**Example: MaleX – 150lbs, 5feet, 32years**

BMR = 66+(6.23x**150**) + (12.7x**60**)-(6.8x**32**)
BMR = 66 + 934.5 + 762 – 217.6
BMR = 1544.9

Assume this short dude works out 4days a week, so his Activity factor is 1.55

newBMR = 1544.9 x **1.55**
newBMR = 2394.6

This means that to maintain his weight, "MaleX" needs to consume 2394 calories a day. So to lose some fat, MaleX obviously needs to eat less than this amount, but the question is *how much* less? I'll discuss this in greater detail in the later chapters when we put everything together.

**The Quick n Dirty BMR Method**

While the Herris-Benedict Formula works well most of the time, there have been times where it was a little off. Based on the number crunching from my clientele data, I've come up with a few constants that I use for a quick and dirty projection of a person's BMR. Here's how it works...

| Activity Level | Bodyweight (lbs) | BMR (calories) |
| --- | --- | --- |
| Low | W | W x 11.5 |
| Medium | W | W x 13.6 |
| High | W | W x 16 |

Now obviously, the value of W will be replaced by your weight. You might be wondering, "If there is such an easy way to calculate your BMR, why go through the trouble of using the formula mentioned earlier?" Well the answer is simple – these values would not exist if it weren't for the formula. The reason I provide two methods is for convenience's sake. The truth is, no BMR calculation will ever be bang on, ever.

There will be those that might misjudge their activity levels and end up consuming more than they need. Others will be too conservative and end up in a caloric deficit. So while the BMR calculations can point you in the right direction, you have to monitor your progress and test it out for yourself.

Think of BMR calculations as the GPS in your car – while it will tell you where to go, you still need to pay attention to your surroundings. Don't be one of those dim-witted doorknobs that ended up driving their car into the lake, and then blamed it on the GPS. Yes, that really happened and makes me slightly fear for our species.

So, take the number you calculated and eat a meal plan based on those numbers for 5 days and monitor your weight. If it stayed the same, you've found your BMR. Spank yourself on the ass for a job well done, or ask your spouse to do so. It's rather motivating. If your weight went up on the other hand, decrease calories by 100-200 and test it again.

If your weight decreased, increase calories by 100 and test again. Don't quit till you've found out how many calories it takes to KEEP you at your weight because once you've found your base, you can start adjusting it to suit your needs.

I guess at this point I should help you choose which method you should use. But I think it's more fun to just let you decide. From my personal experience, people who are generally active tend to do better with the Harris-Benedict formula where as those that don't lift weights and just perform general jogging/leisure sports are better off with the quick and dirty method. Whatever method you decide to go with, be prepared to test out the results.

Now we need to consider another important factor when trying to burn fat - the *quality* of the calories you consume, which brings me to law number two...

**Fat Loss Law #2: Macronutrient Ratios**

**Dialing In The Ratios**

Now that you know what macronutrients are and what your BMR needs to be, we are going to divide up your total daily calories into ratios that will help you lose fat like you wouldn't believe. After testing a shit load of different ratios on my friends, clients, random hamsters, my pet snail, and myself, I have listed a few that have worked quite well. Here they are:

**55P/20C/25F**
**50P/35C/15F**
**45P/30C/25F**
**45P/35C/20F**
**35P/40C/25F**

Each number represents a percentage of your total calories and the corresponding letter represents the type of nutrient.

Using the first ratio as an example, we see that 55% of your daily calories will come from protein, then 20% from carbs and 25% from fats. Now you might be wondering which ratio you should use, so let me shed some light on this. If you're currently on, or know what it's like to go on a low carbohydrate diet, then I highly recommend the first ratio.

It provides the fastest results and allows a bit of leniency towards foods that are slightly higher in fat. However, if you are a total newbie then I suggest you start with ratio #5 and then work your way up. It shouldn't take more than 2-4 weeks to get used to eating with these ratios.

Once you've picked your ratio, it's time to learn how to turn grams into calories. For example, let's say that your BMR is 2000 calories a day... and you ate 100g of carbs, what % is that? Luckily it's all damn easy to calculate. Here's how it works...

**Protein is worth 4 calories per gram**
**Carbs are worth 4 calories per gram**
**Fat is worth 9 calories per gram**

So if you ate 100g of carbs, it would mean you took in 400 calories (100x4).
Now turn that into a percentage: (400/2000) x 100 = 20%

Therefore 20% of your intake was carbs if your BMR is 2000. If you were following ratio #1, you would stop eating carbs at this point. Again, this caloric math might seem lame but fear not, it will soon become second nature. I'll also show you an easier way to handle everything. For now, you just need to have a grasp of the basics.

On a side note, it might be comforting to know that I have E-Training clients who can now eyeball their ratios and most of the time they are bang-on. The hardest part about having a precise eating plan is to get the numbers right.

The first few days might be tedious and you might get a wiff of what it feels like to be an accountant... but just remember that you are handling the wealth of *your* body. If you want stellar results, then you'll have to put in a bit of initial work. Suck it up and deal with it. Things will get easier.

**Tips On Tracking Ratios**

Anyone who says that tracking macronutrient ratios is not feasible for the long term is either:
**a**) a complete idiot
**b**) has never tried this method and doesn't know the benefits it provides or
**c**) has tried, but lacks even the slightest level of discipline and self-respect to stick to it

So don't listen to the losers who couldn't accomplish anything; they usually bark louder than those who were successful. To help you ease into a plan where we track the ratios, I have a few tips that will make the process easier.

**First tip** is to use the Meal Plan Templates in Chapter 7. Get yourself a separate file folder, print them out and get crackin!

**Second tip** is to use a cell phone. At the time of this writing, I own a Galaxy Nexus (which, I might add is *the* shit!) and being a smart phone, it has a boat load of features, one if which is a notepad app where I jot down everything I put in my mouth along with its carb, fat and protein content. Here's an example of what I'd enter:

Sat June 5th 2010
10am 4 egg omlet w/ mixed veggies (32/5/20)

The numbers at the end represent protein, carbs and fats in grams, respectively. If I don't know the macronutrient content of the food, I just write down what I ate and try my best to come up with the numbers later.

You don't have to be *exact*, just close enough. And honestly, how long does it take to jot down one note right before you eat? Actually I timed it. With my cell-phone typing speed, that little entry only took me 25.6 seconds. You're telling me you can't take less than half a minute to write down what you ate? Get real!

**Third tip** is a tiny paper notepad because I get it... not everyone can afford the latest and greatest smart phone (although even the most obsolete cell phones should have a note pad function!) I have clients who buy tiny little notepads with an accompanying tiny pen and it fits right in their pocket. What they do is either carry around the note pad itself or they tear a piece of paper out at the beginning of their day, fold it and toss it in their wallets with the tiny pen. Brilliant!

**A fourth** tip is that you can always talk. Most cell phones (and some mp3 players) have a built-in mic which allows you to record voice recordings and then re-cap everything when you get home. You can even buy tiny, inexpensive voice reminders for under $20.

**Fifth tip** is known as, Evernote. While all the above mentioned tips work just fine, this software is by far the easiest and most "techie" method of keeping track of everything (including your workouts). The process is simple; goto Evernote.com and sign up for a free account. Then you create 2 notebooks, one called "Meal Logs" and another called "Workout Logs". Then, anytime you put anything in your mouth, you create a new "note" in the Meal Log section, throw in any details you might have and be done with it.

Sounds simple, but the magic is in its automation. You don't have to write down the date, the time or any of that extra info because Evernote auto time/date stamps every note. You can literally have hundreds of notes in your Meal Log section and on each one you can see exactly when (and if you choose, where) you ate what you ate. Even better, you can throw in pictures in case you're at a restaurant to keep a more detailed record.

But it gets better. Evernote is what is known as a "cloud" service and therefore, your data can be accessed from anywhere in the world. All you need is an internet connection or a cell reception. You can access Evernote using their free software for your computer, their web-based online software or through an app using your smart phone. All FREE! Is there a catch? Yeah, there is a 60mb/month limit but honestly... I've never gone over 30mb/month and I use Evernote for almost everything such as receipts, notes, thoughts, ideas and my usual fitness data.

And finally there's a **sixth tip** which is so dead simple and genius, I wish I came up with it. Unfortunately though, it was an accidental find on Pinterest[3-15] and I call it "weight loss jars". What you do is get two tiny, clear glass jars. Label one of them "pounds to go" and another one "pounds lost". Then select the amount of weight you want to use (let's say 15) and buy that many colored marbles. Toss these marbles in the "pounds to go" jar and every time you drop a pound, you take one of the marbles and toss them in the "pounds lost" jar. It's simple, effective and very visual way to see your progress, which is why I think it's fucking brilliant.

At this point you really have no excuse. Track everything! Ninety percent of the time when you aren't seeing results, the fault can be spotted and fixed by looking at the logs.

**Fat Loss Law #3: Intense Workouts!**

Obviously, the final law of fat loss is to get your ass moving. Now when it comes to getting ripped, were talking about a very specific type of training regimen. None of that running around for hours or clowning around on the elliptical like a chump. The workouts I prescribe will always accomplish two goals:

1. **Elevate Heart Rate** – This means short rest periods and big compound movements. Throw all the isolation exercises and low intensity cardio out the window.

Isolation exercises are meant to add detail to your physique, which can be done once you've lost a substantial amount of fat. No one is going to notice your biceps if they're adorably wrapped in a layer of fat, get what I'm saying?

2. **Deplete Muscle Glycogen** – Why? To improve insulin sensitivity and use fat in the blood stream as fuel (more on this later). So how do we achieve this? By using free weights that get heavier ever few sessions so that intensity is maximized. Resistance training is *the* way to go when you want to burn fat and keep/build muscle. Some of you might be wondering if resistance bands can be used instead of free weights, and the answer is "yes-no". There are some exercises that just *need* free weights, but most others can be substituted by bands, so working out at home is a definite possibility.

Where does that leave cardio? It leaves it hanging for a very specific time and purpose. The traditional way to workout goes as follows: Hit the gym, warm up, do an hour of weights then do an hour of cardio and leave. Hmm... not only does that take two friggin' hours, it's also pretty inefficient. If you are going to do a *very intense* and short bout of cardio, such as sprints (20 mins or less) after resistance training, fine.

But everything else is not necessary. In fact, those 20 mins shouldn't even be called cardio, more like 'pretending to run from the po-po's as if you just robbed a bank'. So, what's the reason behind not doing cardio after weight training?

Well when you work out with weights at a high intensity, you are training your muscles to become bigger, stronger and use glucose for fuel as efficiently as possible. You're telling them to use up every gram that is available to deliver maximum power in the shortest amount of time. Now when you switch to low intensity cardio and run for an hour, you are signaling your muscles to do the opposite - be as energy efficient as possible (use the least amount of glucose for the required output).

As you can probably tell by now, this is a massive contradiction. It hampers results[3-8] and the only benefit you get out of this type of training is the net calories burnt... which is obviously higher because you're moving around for an extra hour. In my opinion though, the payoff isn't worth the effort.

# Importance Of Insulin Control

Most people think of insulin as the injections that diabetics need to take to prevent themselves from dropping dead. That's true. But there's a lot more to it than that. First we need to know what insulin actually is, and the official description reads like so: *"Insulin is a hormone secreted by the beta cells of the pancreas in response to increased blood levels of glucose and facilitates uptake of glucose by body cells" [J.Thompson, M.Manore, J.Sheeshka, Nutrition - a functional approach].*

Hmm, try saying that to someone the next time you're at a bar and see if they sound impressed. In plain English then, insulin is a hormone that is created in the pancreas and released into the bloodstream when there is a presence of sugar in your blood and it helps stuff all that sugar into cells (such as muscle, or fat).

When it comes to fitness, insulin is basically known as a "storage" hormone. It's kind of like a crazy party chick who is about to go on a vacation; she just loves to stuff her bags to the brim... and if you argue with her about it, you'll lose. Having high levels of insulin then, is a bitch[3-1]!

Furthermore, just like any bitch, insulin can either be your best friend or your worst nightmare (there *are* times where we will spike insulin just as there *are* times where having a bitch on your side is complimentary... more on that later). Now in order for you to burn fat, it must first be released from the fat cells (lipolysis). Only then can it can enter the blood stream as FFA's (free fatty acids) and be used as fuel.

But constantly high levels of insulin will inhibit lipolysis... which means you won't be able to get ripped, no one will like you and you'll probably feel like an unaccomplished loser. We need to avoid this at all costs! So it is of upmost importance that we keep our insulin levels controlled and on the down low.

Now the question is, how exactly does one go about doing that? Easy - by knowing which type of carbohydrates to eat and in what quantities. Having read about the glycemic index in Chapter 2, you should already know which type of carbohydrates will help you achieve low and stable insulin levels.

And my 2nd law of Fat Loss already gave you some effective macronutrient breakdowns so you should be able to put 2 and 2 together. Do you see how all of this comes together so seamlessly? Yeah I know, I make it look too easy.

Also note that when we discuss the advanced Carb Cycling technique, I'll dive into the whole "quantity" aspect of carb intake at a much deeper level. But not *too* deep, this isn't yourporn.com, after all.

# The 3 Stages Of Fat Loss

The process of fat loss, to me, is just like playing an old-school video game where you have stages that get harder and harder as you proceed. Luckily though, fat loss only has 3 stages and if you screw up along the way, you won't have to start from the very beginning. Each of the stages of fat loss refer to the type of fat which you'll be getting rid of - subcutaneous fat (stage 1), visceral fat (stage 2) and stubborn fat (stage 3). Let's talk about the easy part first.

## Stage 1: Subcutaneous Fat

Subcutaneous refers to all the fat that is underneath your skin. If you've ever seen someone with cellulite, than this is what I'm talking about. Not all of subcutaneous fat is bad though, because some is needed as a cushion to protect your body against bumps and other random shit you might walk into on a Friday night, drunk walking with friends. The good news is that subcutaneous fat is the easiest to get rid of when you start the fat loss process. The bad news is that you have no control over how much of it you'll lose. Why? Because it comes down to your genetics... and everyone is a bit different.

Whenever I tell my E-Training clients about the 3 stages of fat loss, the question that always comes up is: "At what point do you go from stage 1 to stage 2 and 3?" and the answer is... I dunno. Again, it's because of the reason I mentioned above – genetics. Your body might like fat under the skin and therefore it'll hang on to it and switch to the next stage earlier than someone else, so you'll just have to see. Speaking of the next stage...

## Stage 2: Visceral Fat

Now visceral fat is a bit harder to get rid of, but definitely not impossible. Not even close.

In fact, just by following my 1st law of fat loss and combining it with adequate training, you can pretty much diminish a shit load of visceral fat. So what is visceral fat? It's the fat that surrounds your internal organs. The good news is that because visceral fat is surrounded by high blood flow, we can get rid of it quickly and efficiently.

Remember, for you to lose fat, you body must first go through the process of lipolysis after which it enters the bloodstream. So if the flow of blood is high around visceral fat, then when the fat is released from the cell, it has an easier time entering the blood stream where we can burn it off. Awesome.

I would say that most people who have 10-12% body fat have successfully completed stage 2, after which they plateau (unless they know what they're doing). This brings us to...

**Stage 3: Stubborn Fat**

To put it simply, stubborn fat is the most annoying shit to get rid of. Have you heard of stories where people say "I was on a diet and it worked for a while, but then I stalled! I just couldn't lose anymore fat! Waaa!" Yeah, what these poor souls experienced was the inability to get rid of stubborn fat. Their so-called diet helped them with stage 1 and 2, but got shut down on stage 3. The sad part is that they will keep trying and will not see any improvements.

This will result in discouragement, which will result in them giving up, which will result in them bouncing back to the weight they were at initially(or higher).

So what exactly makes stubborn fat so damn stubborn? Well the first reason is the exact opposite of what makes visceral fat (fairly) easy to get rid of – blood flow.

Generally, stubborn fat is stored around the gut (love handles), lower back, triceps (flabby arm syndrome) and the thighs.

And as you can probably guess, these sites in your body have abysmal blood circulation. So even if you *can* get your body to release the fat from these stubborn deposit spots, there is no guarantee it will enter the bloodstream and be used as fuel. In fact, in most cases it will just go right back into the fat cell (known as re-esterfication). How bad does that suck? Pretty damn bad.

Another reason why stubborn fat is challenging is because it does not respond to adrenal hormones (adrenaline and noradrenaline) as well as visceral fat. And why are adrenal hormones important? Because they trigger fat burnnanation! (Erm, it's technically called fat oxidation... but that doesn't sound nearly as cool). Now add these two reasons on top of each other and it almost makes you want to give up on fat loss - but don't you dare!

You see, we have two secret weapons called **Carb Cycling** and **Ass Busting Training Routines**, and their specific job is to help you blast away stubborn fat. You can also use fasting (**ifast**) as another weapon, should you choose to use it. And if you really want to get even with your love handles, there are a few supplements and compounds which will further help turn the tide of sexiness in your favor.

# On Fasting

Intermittent Fasting (from now on, referred to as "ifast") has become all the rage these days, and as such, I've gotten countless emails asking me about my thoughts on this method. Well here they are: *Useful When Needed!*

I'll admit it, I used to think ifast was kind of retarded. There were a few reasons for this - first and foremost, I and plenty of others have managed to achieve a model-like physique without the need to resist food for long ass periods of time. I had a plan which worked, allowed me to eat filling foods and even out-right cheat on the weekends. Second, fasting was usually an option for those that had food sensitivities and therefore needed to go on elimination diets or detox diets.

And finally, all ifast really does is provide a (convenient?) way to accomplish one of the universal laws of fat loss - caloric restriction. The HGH increases and all the other touted "benefits" can be achieved by lifting heavy loads against gravity coupled with a low carb diet... so it's all marketing ammo as far as I'm concerned. What's more, low calorie diets can essentially do what fasting does, and that is increase blood flow to the fat cells, which allows a greater chance of burning fat as fuel.

If there's one thing I know, it's that 99% of human beings *like* to eat on some level and *do not* like the feeling of hunger, so when ifast started to pick up steam, I was rather baffled. As they say, the truth is in the pudding... mmm pudding. I suggest you read *Eat Stop Eat* (fitjerk.com/eatstopeat) by Brad Pilon. But what made ifast *really* interesting is a dude named Martin Berkhan.

Martin shrunk down the fasting times to 16 hours and played around with the protocol till his clients were seeing favorable results - which really made me take notice.

It was after this real-world proof that I decided to experiment with ifast protocols with clients that wanted to give it a shot. Overall results were positive.

Scientific reasons aside, the reason ifast works well is because there is not much thinking involved. You starve yourself...err, I mean "fast" for a certain amount of hours, then you break the fast and eat your required calories during the "feeding" time frame within 2-3 meals. Speaking of meal frequency, there was a study[3-2] done, where they took sixteen obese individuals and fed them either 3 meals + 3 snacks or just 3 outright meals per day for 8 weeks. Here's what they found...

*"...there were no significant differences between the low- and high-MF groups for adiposity indices, appetite measurements or gut peptides (peptide YY and ghrelin) either before or after the intervention. We conclude that increasing MF (meal frequency) **does not** promote greater body weight loss under the conditions described in the present study."*

So physiologically, eating frequent meals is irrelevant when it comes to fat loss. However, psychologically it can be a different story (more on that later).

**Who Should Consider ifast?**

I usually recommend ifast to clients who are extremely busy and don't have much time to devote to a fine-tuned plan or those that have achieved their desired body and want to maintain it for the rest of their life. It's also for those that don't have a nasty snacking habit and don't feel much pain or discomfort when they go without food for long ass periods of time.

Take someone who works 12 hour office shifts on the daily – this person probably wakes up at 6am, goes to work at 7am and doesn't come home till 7pm.

During their work shift, this person will usually get an hour for lunch and maybe a tiny break where they will end up buying garbage food that is very calorie dense, leading to weight gain over a period of time. Assuming they sit on their ass all day, of course.

But if they were on an ifast protocol which was in sync with their daily routine, they would fast from 2am – 6pm (16 hours), and this way not have to worry about eating during work. He/She can just have a coffee and relax. They can worry about other, more important things in life such as whether or not their favorite contestant will get kicked off Dancing With The Stars tonight... or whatever the hell it is that people watch these days.

Here's where ifast shines: Since the feeding time for this theoretical person starts at 7pm, their dinner can be as big as they want because realistically, they probably have to hit the sack by 12am. This leaves them with 5 hours to eat an entire day's worth of calories – which will most likely not happen. And even if it does, it's very unusual for them to go OVER their maintenance (BMR) unless they're a ridiculous pig of an eater.

If you want to try ifast, below are a few structured protocols for you. Ifast can be as complicated or as simple as you want it to be. The fasting portion is easy, but when it comes to feeding, you can either "just eat" or calculate your caloric needs, figure out your maco ratios and pick specific foods to help with recovery or fat loss.

**The Simple Method (From *Eat Stop Eat*)**
**Step 1:** Don't eat for a 24 hour period
**Step 2:** Err... that's about it.

Yep, it's really *that* simple. Pick any 24 hour period – 6pm to 6pm or 9pm to 9pm etc. and don't eat. Then once the fast is over, eat! You can do 1-3 of these sessions per week. Water, coffee and tea are allowed.

What will really blow your mind is how there are entire video and audio courses that cost half a Benjamin and take hundreds of hours to explain what I did in three measly sentences. Can you say power to the people?

Alright, that's just one of the fasting protocols and it works, but the one I recommend for most people (specially guys that want to optimize muscle mass) is the 16 hour fast followed by the 8 hour feed as outlined in the 12 hour worker example. Unlike the 24 hour fast though, I recommend you fine tune what you put in your mouth during the feeding period by figuring out your maintenance calories and then adjusting them to fit your needs (more on this later in the book).

## The Advanced Method

**Step 1:** Figure out when you want to take your 16 hour fast. Once you decide on your fasting time, it's crucial you don't change it. The reason is that you want your body to get used to this protocol, and constantly changing your shit around will equal fat loss doom. So think hard, but don't hurt yourself. A solid suggestion is to structure your fast while you work so you don't have to worry about food. It's what smart people do. But you can be dumb too, it's cool - the plan will work either way.

**Step 2:** Figure out your maintenance caloric requirement. This can be done using the Harris Benedict Formula or the Quick n Dirty BMR Method in my *"Three Golden Laws Of Fat Loss"* section.

*If fondling raw numbers isn't your thing and you bought the digital PRO version of this book, then make use of the calculator that was included. (If you'd like to upgrade to the PRO version, email me your amazon receipt and I'll send you the upgrade link)*

**Step 3:** Reduce the BMR number from step2 by 15% Do you really need an explanation for this step? I sure as hell hope not.

**Step 4:** Figure out your macro ratios
Now that you know how many calories you need to take in during your feed, you should spend some time and divide up your calories into ratios that you want (the attached calculator will do this for you). This should give you exactly how many grams of protein, carbs and fats you should eat. As a rule of thumb, don't drop protein below 30% - that's the bare minimum.

**Step 5:** Create the meal plan
Based on the numbers you now have, create a meal plan which you'll use during your 8 hour feeding window.

**A few things to remember**

First, make sure you don't do your workouts (especially resistance training) in a fasted state because you'll probably compromise muscle mass. Structure your plan so that when you break your fast, it happens to be a pre-workout meal. A protein shake with an adequate amount of carbs is an excellent pre-workout meal/fast breaker.

Consume *most* of your carbs and calories post workout. The reason is simple - muscle glycogen levels are low after you've been lifting so your body will soak up all the calories you throw at it. Assuming your intensity was above average, your metabolic rate should also be on fire, so it's the perfect time to eat.

Avoid carb heavy meals before bed time. If you followed the tip above, then this bullet point should be a non-issue. Unless of course you workout late at night, and in that case it doesn't matter. No point in losing sleep over a carb issue. Carbophobia is very real, potatoes have been known haunt people's dreams. Don't fall for such a trap.

If you are a dude (or dudette) who is looking to add muscle mass while simultaneously trying to lose the fat, ignore step 3 and monitor your body fat levels.

If anything, you might need to increase your calories that you take in. Don't add 500 right away - for lean mass gains that's too big of a jump. Start with increments of 100 and track, track, track. Get to know the body fat caliper as well as your right hand during those lonely Friday nights.

Back to fat loss - if after 2-3 weeks you aren't losing weight, don't freak out and spam me with your ridiculous emails. First, check to make sure that your body fat levels are dropping. The scale may not show much improvement, but if your jeans fit looser, you're making progress. If you're totally convinced the plan isn't working, drop your calories by 200 and monitor for another week. Keep doing this still you start to lose weight.

**Why Fasting Seems To Work**

While the ifast protocol is pretty straight forward and simple, the reason I believe it *really* works is because our bodies are most likely meant to eat in such a way.

I usually make fun of Paleo dieters because they talk my ears off about what our ancestors ate, why it's super important and all that other hoopla. However, the focus should be on *how & when* they ate their food. If you lived in a caveman tribe, you didn't have food available to you on demand like you do today. No drive-throughs or deliveries. Bummer. So if you wanted food, you had to grow some balls, pick up a spear (or a rock if you were the technologically challenged caveman) and go hunt a wild buffalo. Or some other equally large and delicious animal.

But, if your hunting session failed, you wouldn't have food till you got up and tried hunting again on another day. Assuming you succeeded on the 2nd day, you would now be able to eat for an entire week. You would have meat when you wanted it, sex when you wanted it (because cave chicks totally dig successful hunters) and sleep when you wanted it. Life would be good.

But alas, after a week it would be time to hunt yet again. And so the cycle of "fasting" and "feeding" went on for hundreds of thousands (or even millions) of years. That's probably the most basic, stripped down and naked explanation I could come up with.

Now if you compare a feeding cycle that went on for something like *millions of years* to modern farming, which has been around for a few thousand years, you quickly get the picture; easily available food is *not* what our bodies are designed for. This is why a majority of the population ends up in a caloric surplus at the end of the day. Resulting in fatter asses, bigger love handles and double chins. How attractive.

Now when you take the ifast protocol, which jives with the way our bodies are used to consuming food, and throw in proper macro ratios along with heavy resistance training, what you have is a recipe for a very lean and sexy physique.

While that theory makes good logical sense, the flip side of the coin is that if you've been eating frequent meals for years (or even decades) your physiology has gotten used to that eating pattern. This is why when you first start ifast (especially if you're an old fart) you'll get hunger pangs that will make you want to punch a new born kitten.

And because I think new born kittens are rather adorable, I don't recommend fasting for older clients. At least not until they're reasonably lean (10-12% BF). They are just too used to eating all the damn time and it's just easier to change up their meal plan then get them to fast.

That's not to say that ifast will be impossible to get used to if you want to give it a real shot. You could get used to it in a week, two weeks or it could take a month. Millions of years worth of evolution can't just vanish because you've been eating frequently for a few decades. Everyone's different, so try it out and see how you feel.

# Leptin – The Ultimate Middle Man

If you read about leptin from a bunch of sources you'll find that some say it's a protein and others call it a hormone. Who's right? To be honest they all are, since leptin is actually a protein hormone. It is located on chromosome 7 in humans and its job is to act as the middleman between what's happening in your body and what your brain *thinks* is happening in your body. Put simply, leptin is a hormone (alongside a bunch of other hormones) that signals the brain about how much fat you have on your ass and how much you're eating.

Now a quick side note - functions in your body such as metabolic rate, appetite and hunger are controlled by certain neurochemicals. The cool (or unfortunate) thing is that the level of leptin in your body directly affects the level of these neurochemicals.

So if your leptin levels drop, your brain will signal these neurochemicals to come out and play, making you feel hungry, decreasing your metabolic rate (so you don't starve to death) and increasing your appetite when your senses pick up the slightest hint of food availability. And when do your leptin levels drop? Well, when you start to diet.

Your "normal" leptin levels are based on your body fat levels. The fatter you are, the more leptin you have and the leaner you are, the less leptin you have. In 1994, they studied an OB (obese) mouse which put on weight extremely easily and had a very low metabolic rate.

As it turns out, this overgrown mouse was defective and produced absolutely zero leptin, which meant that it was probably hungry all the damn time and couldn't stop eating. To see what effect leptin would have on this fat rodent, they injected it with synthetic leptin and lo-behold, it started to lose weight at a rapid pace.

So a rise in leptin levels trigged a neurochemical response to decrease hunger, appetite and increase the rat's resting metabolic rate.

Now I know what you're thinking, "Screw exercise, I'll just stick leptin needles in my ass and voila!" Sadly, it's not that damn simple. First of all, synthetic leptin is absurdly expensive - we're talking thousands of dollars. Second, increasing leptin levels beyond what's considered "normal" by your body doesn't really seem to have much of an effect as much as lowering leptin does because of something called leptin resistance.

The higher your leptin levels, the more resistant you are to it. The mouse was a special case, it had none to begin with so a synthetic shot did it some good. You're not so lucky. There go your dreams of being a leptin injecting junkie. If it makes you feel any better, you could give the thousands you were thinking of spending to me.

So ultimately, what is the point of you knowing about leptin? So you can go impress your date at the bar tomorrow night? Hardly. (Although, saying that your leptin levels are lower than the average population might get a bio nerd rather wet.) Understanding leptin allows you fundamentally understand why potent/hardcore diets *cannot* be long term solutions to fat loss.

They are like exotic sports cars; they'll get you to your destination with flare and speed but fail at being the practical, long-term family vehicle. It doesn't matter how good your will power is, extreme dieting *without* proper re-feeds and breaks will lead to lower than normal leptin levels which will always make your body crave food.

However, there is an odd phenomenon that occurs when people use ifast as their diet/weight loss strategy. We know that lowering calories (dieting) will lead to weight loss and lowered leptin levels, but what about when you cut off food all together for short periods of time? Well, it turns out you lose weight but *without* the reduction in your leptin levels.

Now, if leptin controls the triggering of neurochemicals that control appetite and hunger, why do you feel hungry when you practice fasting? You leptin levels haven't dropped, so what gives? The answer is simple: during a fast, those neurochemicals that activate hunger get triggered regardless of your leptin levels. It's as if all of a sudden, they have a mind of their own.

Let's connect a few more dots:

If dieting = drop in leptin levels, which = increase in hunger...

and ifast = no drop in leptin levels, but still = increase in hunger...

Why bother fasting at all? Well first and foremost, ifast may just be a more convenient option for you as I explained in the fasting section. But physiologically it could be a superior option due to the fact that leptin promotes fat oxidation (burning) in your muscles and spares glucose. So *not* having it drop could be a good thing.

So if you're keen on holding on to your muscle mass, keeping your leptin levels normal is a good idea. But while your leptin levels will drop during carb cycling (since it's a "diet"), you will also get cheat days where you eat a bucket load of food, bouncing those levels back up and putting you in a state of anabolism. So don't fret.

**The Wrap Up**

If you're a complete newbie to the world of dieting and fat loss, then that was probably a mouthful of info to digest all in one go. As a result, I've summarized everything about leptin as well as thrown in some extra fun facts below... in case you're feeling extra nerdy today.

Leptin is a protein hormone and the "normal" amount in your body depends on how much fat you have. Lean people = low leptin, fat people = more leptin.

Change in leptin levels have a direct impact on the neurochemicals that influence hunger, appetite and metabolism.

When leptin levels drop below your normal range, your body will fire up the hunger machine. When leptin levels rise, the reverse happens, without overcompensation.

The more leptin you have, the more resistant you are to it. Leptin is produced by fat cells and the amount produced depends on the amount of glucose you have in you. Low glucose levels (dieting) impedes production while a glucose surplus (eating) increases it.

You cannot sustain low leptin levels (diets) for a long period of time without feeling like shit, therefore cheat days where leptin levels can get a boost, are necessary.

An ifast protocol allows you to achieve a weekly caloric deficit without dropping your leptin levels, however the hunger pangs will still exist since the neurochemicals will still be triggered. Leptin can promote fat oxidation in fat cells and make them resistant to insulin. This is a good thing since we know that insulin is a storage hormone.

A decrease in leptin also interferes with your body's immune response time, therefore taking precautions against getting colds is a MUST when trying to get extremely lean (single digit body fat levels.)

So there you have it, my attempt at simplifying the explanation of leptin for the masses. I think if I simplified it any more, I'd get hate mail from the nerds.

# Paleo Or Mayo?

Eating Paleo* is another one of those trends that has become hot these days, and as such, people are following this trend without putting an ounce of thought into the process. It's like high-school all over again; people are doing it because everyone else is doing it. Sometimes, the human race is such a mindless group of sheep, I tell ya.

Fortunately I'm a wolf, and therefore I will help you answer the major question that's burning up your insides: *"Should I or should I not follow a Paleo diet?"*

In my opinion, it all comes down to energy levels and not "health benefits". What I've observed is that a major part of our population hasn't yet adapted to foods such as grains, oats etc. Sure we can eat them, but we humans have been consuming fruits, plants and meat for way longer. This means we can digest them better and faster. Don't believe me? Just take a look at the stats:

The potato was introduced to Europe by Spain around the 1500's. But as far as consumption goes, I'd say our actual exposure to potatoes ranges anywhere from 3000-5000 years. Maybe slightly more.

Now compare that to meat and plants which our ancestors have been consuming for the better part of millions of years and it's not hard to see why our population hasn't fully adapted yet. Give it another 10,000-20,000 years and the Paleo diet will be thing of the, er... past?

So how do you know if your body is adept at breaking down these "New Age Carbs"? Simple, you test it out just like you did when we talked about food combination. After you wake up and take a shower, predict your current energy level and write it down using a scale of 1-10. Just make an educated guess if you aren't sure.

Then, follow this up with a full featured, carb heavy breakfast. It should consist only of new age carbs, so something like a bagel, some pancakes and lots of syrup. Try not to ingest anything else such as stimulants (caffeine) during this experiment.

After about an hour or so, see how you feel and write down your energy level again on a scale of 1-10. If your post-meal energy level remained the same or increased, then congratulations, you can handle New Age Carbs just fine and don't need to follow the Paleo type lifestyle. If however you are like me, and find yourself passing the fuck out on the couch from such a carb-heavy meal then New Age Carbs are something you're going to have to limit. **Hint:** Not eliminate. Why?

The reason is that whole wheat, oats and bunch of other New Age Carbs are Low Glycemic, which means they have their uses. Also, in this day and age it's almost impossible to live a Paleo lifestyle 24/7. It's more cumbersome than beneficial... though it can be done if you try *extra* hard.

Screw that.

* For those who find themselves asking the question, "FJ, what's a Paleo Diet?" Here's the official description from thepaleodiet.com:

"The Paleo Diet is a way of eating in the modern age that best mimics diets of our hunter-gatherer ancestors - combinations of lean meats, seafood, vegetables, fruits, and nuts.

By eating the foods that we are genetically adapted to eat, followers of the Paleo Diet are naturally lean, have acne-free skin, improved athletic performance, and are experiencing relief from numerous metabolic-related and autoimmune diseases."

*It basically means that if cavemen didn't eat it or couldn't safely consume it, then you shouldn't either. The Paleo dieter shuns things like grains, wheat, under-ground vegetables such as carrots and potatoes etc. I call these "New Age Carbs" because they've only been around for the better part of a few thousand years. Consequently, "Old Age Carbs" were anything that a caveman could safely access and consume.*

# Meal & Nutrition Timing

As if knowing how much you should eat daily isn't enough, the next "technique" most health gurus seem to verbally vomit is the idea of *when* to eat. Some say pre workout, some say post workout, some say eat a lot in the morning and some say eat everything in the evening.

Who is right? Does this amount of anal retentiveness even matter? The answer isn't as black and white as you might want it to be, but the implementation is pretty damn simple.

First of all, <u>nothing</u> is more important than your total macronutrient intake by the end of the day. It doesn't matter if you ate a salad post workout, stuffed your face during breakfast, had no lunch, or pigged out before bed time. As long as you hit your macronutrient requirements before you get some shut eye, you'll be ahead of 95% of the population.

When it comes to my clients, I want to keep things as stupidly easy as possible and so what I do, is make them a meal plan and tell them they can eat the foods however and whenever they wish, as long as they don't eat anything extra by the time they end up in bed. Seems to be working rather well, if I should say so myself.

Another advantage of this approach is that the stick ratio is high since it allows them to carry on with their normal life without worrying about when to eat. Now, there was a study[3-3] done in 1997 which took 10 women, divided them into two groups (AM group and a PM group) and fed them two meals per day; breakfast and lunch. For 6 weeks straight, the AM group ate about 70% of their daily calories during breakfast while the PM group obviously took in their 70% during the evening.

After the 6 weeks were up, they swapped the groups so now the AM group became the PM group, and the PM group became the AM group and did the whole morning/evening shebang for another 6 weeks.

At the end of the 15 week study (3 weeks were used as a stabilization period), the results were rather interesting. On average, the AM group lost more weight than the PM group, however the PM group lost more *fat mass* than the AM group. Basically, those that ate a heavy breakfast and a light dinner ended up losing fat as well as muscle mass, but those that ate light in the mornings but heavy in the evenings lost mainly fat.

The take home point is that if you have control over when you eat your meals, you are better off stuffing your face at night, since we're looking to get ripped, not just thin. However if you can't, don't sweat you pink little panties because your body composition will improve due to proper resistance training, where as the subjects in the study were prescribed training routines that I would call "pathetic" at best.

Their exercise subscription consisted of three elements: walking, aerobics (such as a treadmill) and a weight training circuit using Universal machines. The only positive thing I saw was the use of progressive overload (lifting heavier weekly). But the simple fact is this: traditional cardio sucks balls and calling the use of Universal machines "weight lifting" is like calling a buger-flipper at McDonald's a Masterchef. It's absurd.

The point I'm trying to make by completely bashing their exercise protocols is that I have a little prediction: If a proper free-weight resistance training program was used, it would have closed the gap between the AM and the PM group, leaving us with what I said above: Don't stress over it. Consume most of your foods in the evening, but only if you have the time to do so.

## Pre and Post Workout Nutrition

Depending on your individual goal, what and how much you take in before your workout tends to differ. But since this book is concerned with fat loss, and our exercise regimen of choice is resistance training, the goal is to minimize muscle protein breakdown while increasing fat oxidation.

First of all, you should know that your pre and post workout meals are not exempt from being included into your daily macronutrient allowance. Second, the type of pre and post workout meal (solid or liquid) will largely depend on the time between ingestion and workout.

If your workout is more than an hour away, I recommend you stick to solid foods. If your workout is 45minutes away or less, bust out that blender because you'll be chugging down a glass off mixed deliciousness.

The next thing we need to tackle is what you should eat (or drink). Should it be protein, carbs, fats... alcohol? This depends on which fat loss plan you are following, and so I have a bunch of different answers:

**1.** If you are following the ifast protocol and you cannot manage to time the fast-breaking meal as your pre-workout meal, then you will need to take one scoop of unflavored whey isolate protein (~28g) with water. Post workout nutrition should ideally be a carbohydrate heavy meal but should also have protein in it. It bears repeating that you should try not to do resistance training in a fasted state.

Now, don't be completely paranoid either; if it's 1pm and time for your workout, but you forgot your protein powder at home, don't skip your damn workout. Do it, then have your fast breaking meal. The world won't come to an end, you'll be fine. In fact, training in a fasted state only affects the duration of your workout, not the intensity.

So you'll be able to go hard, but for not as long (I hear you perform similarly in the bedroom anyways, so no big deal). A scoop of protein powder before your workout is the most ideal scenario... but sometimes, life happens, so go with it.

**2.** If you are following the carbohydrate cycling plan (more on that soon), then you'll again take one scoop whey protein isolate (~28g) with water before your depletion workouts. The only difference is that you may use protein shakes which are flavored (i.e., have 10g or less sugar for added taste). For your cardio workouts... it doesn't really matter, just eat something from your meal plan before and after.

For your weekend strength workouts, eat a balanced protein and carb meal beforehand, along with another balanced protein and carb meal after. An example would be to have 3 eggs and 2 slices of toast 45-60 minutes prior, followed by a chicken breast, veggies and a glass of juice post workout.

**3.** If you are following a general calorie deficit plan then my ideal suggestion is to take a scoop of whey protein isolate 30 minutes before your workout followed by a significantly solid meal (30-50% of your calories) post workout with a balanced protein/carb ratio. It doesn't get much simpler than that.

I think you're starting to see a general trend here, and that is you should "sandwich" your workouts with protein and/or protein + carbs. Why? Because you'll not only build muscle and get stronger, but help facilitate a slightly greater rate of fat loss then if you didn't[3-10].

Finally, if you cannot manage to take anything pre-workout, post-workout or both, then don't stress it. It all comes back full circle to the main point I made earlier – as long as your macronutrient ratios are met before bed time, you'll be fine.

# Advanced Carb Cycling

I have a love/hate relationship with this technique. I love it because it works faster than almost anything else out there (besides the help of illegal pharmaceuticals) and lets me stuff my face over the weekends. However, I hate it because during the week the workouts coupled with low calorie food intake is straight up - no other way to put it - a complete bitch and a half.

You'll feel tired and you'll hate yourself for a brief period of time, so don't say I didn't warn you. That said we do have a valiant tool on our side – caffeine. It should keep you going till the weekend, where you can let all hell break loose.

## Why It Works – Psychologically

I'll be the first to say it – the caloric deficit that you must endure over the weekdays is not sustainable for the long term. This is why carb cycling is a short-term, advanced strategy that you should use to "fine tune" your aesthetics rather than use it as the primary technique to lose fat. But, the lure of the weekend carb load (also known as re-feed or cheat day) pretty much carries you through the week. A nice benefit is that the caloric requirements for the weekends are so high, that you'll practically be forced to eat "junk."

Want burgers? Done. Want ice cream? Done. Want chocolate? Can't have me. Best of all I can honestly say, hand on balls, that I have never managed to go through a carb loading day without having to resort to caloric dense, junk foods. It's just too uncomfortable to eat "clean" foods in order to meet the requirements. And the best part out of all of this? Eating junk doesn't really have a negative effect on results, assuming you stay on course with your macro ratios of course.

When clients are on a regular deficit plan, I tell them to make a dream list of foods that they would want to eat on their cheat days. I allow them to throw in whatever the hell they want as long as the list isn't absurdly long (stick to 3-5).

After reaching their goal weight, I'll throw them on the carb cycling plan to drop their body fat percentages even lower and create a cheat-day meal plan by throwing in (almost) everything they listed on their dream list. It's a solid way to motivate them to work on their current plan so that in the future they can look forward to their ~~cheat~~ carb loading days. I suggest you do the same.

Take out a piece of paper and write down all the junk foods that will satisfy your cravings and make sure that list isn't more than five items long. This will ensure that you'll take in a huge quantity of the foods you love, resulting in overcompensation (you won't want to eat them again till the next weekend.) They say too much of anything can be bad... and we kinda want to follow the same principle.

If you love pizza and just eat a few slices over the weekend, chances are that you'll want it again during the weekdays. On the other hand, if you stuff your face with more pizza than Michaelangelo from the Ninja Turtles, chances are you'll not want to look at another slice till next weekend.

## Why It Works – Physiologically

First of all, when you reduce the amount of food that goes into you (a caloric deficit), your blood glucose drops. Which makes sense - if you're eating less, you're probably taking in less carbohydrates. As such, your insulin levels drop as well. Recall that insulin is a storage hormone - so if there isn't much to store, then it isn't needed. It would be like hiring 20 guys to help you move a few boxes of office junk down the street. Completely un-necessary.

When these two situations occur, it allows for fat to be mobilized from the fat cells and it enters into your bloodstream to (hopefully) be used as fuel, since carbohydrates (the primary fuel source) is scarce. The fat is then burnt off by your tissues and organs. Sounds nice, doesn't it?

Unfortunately, that isn't enough (as anyone who has tried any type of diet in the past knows). While it's true that a regular caloric deficit will help you drop weight, you need to undergo glycogen (sugar) depletion in your muscles to really use all of the fat in your blood stream as fuel. But the problem is that your muscles will not let go of the glycogen that they've already stored within. They cling on to it like a scared toddler grabs on to their mother's hand.

So if your muscles are already filled with glycogen (their primary source of fuel), why would they use the fat in the blood stream as another fuel source? It makes no sense. Think of it this way: regardless of how much a fat kid loves cake, you cannot feed him more if he is full; his eyes might say "yes" but his bodily functions say "no".

So on one hand, you need glycogen depletion to maximize beta oxidation (the burning of fat as fuel) but on the other, you need to get rid of your current glycogen stores first ("empty the tank" sort to speak).

How do we do this?

**Easy - lift heavy ass weights.**

Lifting results in your muscles expending the stored glycogen as fuel and once this fuel source runs out, they have no choice but to use the fat in your blood stream to keep going. And keep going you will, because that bar on the rack ain't gona squat itself.

This brings us to the next point. If all you have to do is "diet" and introduce some resistance training, what the hell is the point of the carb load? Why can't you just keep on doing this forever, or at least until you end up with a body that makes people get random heart palpitations?

And the answer is simple: along with the good, there is also the bad. While dropping calories to a level I'll be recommending allows you to use fat as a fuel source, it also drops your leptin levels (which as you may recall, tells your brain that you aren't eating and results in hunger pangs) and increases cortisol levels which *can* result in protein breakdown.

Your immune function will also start to suffer when you go on such a deficit for a long period of time. So what we do is after a few days of ~~hell~~ reducing calories, we introduce a huge carb load (or re-feed). What this does it the exact opposite of everything you just read. Leptin levels go back to normal, cortisol levels drop, protein synthesis (building of new muscle) increases, hunger pangs go away and you feel like a rock-star that just got swarmed by a horde of sweaty groupies.

What's more, if you stick to the carb load cycle I recommend, you'll hardly gain any fat. So really, it's the best of both worlds. You just have to put in the work.

## Training On Low Calories

If you've been around the "fitness scene" sort to speak, and your primary goal is to make sure you don't lose an ounce of muscle which you've worked hard for, then the low carb days will make you slightly uneasy. The common concern is, *"won't I lose all the hard earned muscle on my body?"* The answer is no.

No you won't.

I used to think that significant muscle loss was a price I'd have to pay to get lean, however I never noticed any significant drop. This was years ago and I never bothered to dig around as to why. Today though, I got me some science to prove it, bro!

There was a study[3-7] done where they took twenty people and fed them 800 calories a day in the form of a liquid diet. These people were separated into 2 groups: A control plus diet (C+D) and a resistance exercise plus diet (R+D). The C+D group were told to perform some weak sauce cardio for an hour a day, four times a week and the R+D group did some form of circuit resistance training (to work the whole body, I presume) while increasing the volume of work done at a progressive rate.

The results put a huge smile on my face. Let me quote, "**The addition of an intensive, high volume resistance training program <u>resulted in preservation of LBW</u> (*Lean* Body Weight) and RMR (Resting Metabolic Rate) during weight loss with a VLCD (Very Low Calorie Diet).**" [bolding mine]

And preservation of lean mass is actually the lowest common denominator, because if your workouts are intelligently designed, you will not only preserve muscle mass, you can increase it *while* improving your strength levels. How do I know? Real world experience and data on my clients, myself and countless other trainers. In fact my Swedish homeboy, Dr.Bojan Kostevski (who wrote the preface to this book) recently did a bonkers low calorie experiment which he coined as ILCD (Insanely Low Calorie Diet).

Basically, the man took a hit of 2000 calories per day, for 6 days straight. All the while still forcing himself to live out a normal, daily life. And as a doctor who walks around decently lean, his "normal daily life" involved work in the ER and hitting up the gym frequently.

Some "experts" considered this insane, and even unhealthy. Or in layman's terms, those that didn't have the sheer balls or willpower to do what he did, started talking smack to get attention. Probably in the hopes that someone, somewhere might consider them important and relevant.

It's no surprise that the process was grueling, and was well documented[3-9]. It also resulted in a pretty substantial transformation (loss of 5lbs in 8 days). While this got most people all wet, I was more intrigued by his performance in the gym and life in general.

Not only did his focus remain strong (kind of important when you're dealing with dying patients in the ER), but his strength actually increased by a shitload (he smashed a few of his personal records). The ending conclusion by Dr.Kostevski was, "how you feel is a lie". Remember that statement when you're hating life due to one of my hardcore workouts.

The bottom line? As long as you bust your behind, lift heavy stuff off the floor and generally avoid being an unflattering chump, muscle loss during a lower calorie eating isn't something you need to be concerned with – assuming you follow smart protocols. You should also take comfort in the fact that my protein recommendations are on the higher end, so that's another fail safe tool you have at your disposal.

# Why The hCG Diet Is For Dimwit Pee-Lovers

*I've gotten countless questions on this ridiculous diet over the past few months and so, it was only fitting that I inform you about this scam machine which seems to be sweeping the nation. What we have below is a piece that was written by **Dr.Bojan Kostevski** (yes, the same man who did the ILCD experiment earlier).*

*Not only is he a talented writer but quite the expert in making diet cheesecakes that look so delicious, you'll have a sudden, uncontrollable urge to lick your screen. So there was no reason for me to verbalize what he had already done so brilliantly.*

So the summer is closing up on us and people start to fantasize about the perfect beach body. How do I know? Because all the spam on my twitter is driving me nuts. A lot of it is advertisement for fat loss products, some more popular than others.

One commonly advertised substance is hCG. Now I've heard of this substance before (not at least while reading obstetrics and gynecology in med school). I decided to look at the claims made for the substance and take a look if there is any scientific backing on the supposed effects of the hCG diet.

### hC-what?

hCG (or human chorionic gonadotrophin) is a hormone produced during the early part of pregnancy and stimulates the production of progesterone and estrogens and is crucial for the development of the placenta. It is the hormone measured in pregnancy tests and is the biochemical indication of a successful pregnancy. hCG injections are derived from female urine and are used in medicine to treat conditions such as infertility due to anovulation, medically assisted reproduction and to treat delayed puberty in boys.

But the question is, why would people inject something derived from urine for fat loss purposes?

## HCG-diet

More than 50 years ago, Dr. Albert T. Simeons, a British endocrinologist published a study[3-4], claiming that HCG injections would enable dieters to subsist comfortably on a 500-calorie-a-day diet. The setup was as follows: a 500-calorie-a-day diet (high protein, low fat/carbs) in combination with daily hCG intramuscular injections that was claimed to:

a. Enhance fat mobilization
b. Suppress appetite
c. Redistribute fat from the waist, hips and thighs
d. Increase overall well-being.

Besides the insanely low caloric intake and daily (brutally painful) injections of the substance, this sounds awesome. And the anecdotal data proves that people who followed the hCG diet really did lose a lot of weight. Awesome.

But was it because of the hCG injections? Hell no.

### Why the HCG-diet *seems* to work

The hCG diet will make you lose weight for sure, but the question is, "can a 500 calorie-a-day diet without the painful injections have the same effect?"

There have been quite a few randomized studies done on the topic and the conclusion is that none of the effects are enhanced with injections of hCG as compared to the 500 calorie diet by itself.

One large meta analysis[3-5] from 1995 looked at the results from 24 different studies on the effects of the hCG diet. The results are summarized in the picture below.

Table 3 Simeons therapy for treatment of obesity; particulars of the available randomised clinical trials

| (First) author [ref.] | Regime† | Loss to follow-up HCG* % | control % | a | b | c | d |
|---|---|---|---|---|---|---|---|
| Stein [29] | standard | 0 | 0 | neg | neg | neg | |
| Young [30] | + lectures on diet and behaviour twice a week | 20 | 10 | neg | neg | | |
| Shetty [31] | standard | 0 | 0 | neg | neg | neg | neg |
| Mens [32] | + daily group sessions | 0 | 0 | neg | | neg | |
| Richter [33] | 250 iu HCG daily, control group got no injections, only diet; weekly supporting interview | 4 | 4 | neg | neg | neg | neg |
| Bosch [23] | + lectures on obesity and behaviour once a week | 15 | 20 | neg | neg | neg | neg |
| Greenway [34] | HCG dose not mentioned | 10 | 35 | neg | neg | neg | neg |
| Asher [35] | standard | 0 | 0 | pos | | | pos |
| | | 0 | 10 | | | pos | |
| Craig [36] | standard | 0 | 0 | neg | | | |
| Richter [33] | all patients used contraceptives; 250 iu HCG daily, control group got no injections, only diet; weekly supporting interview | 13 | 6 | neg | neg | neg | neg |
| Miller [37] | standard | 0 | 0 | neg | | neg | neg |
| Frank [38] | 1030 kcal. daily + 3 times weekly 200 iu HCG subcutaneously | 0 | 0 | neg | neg | neg | neg |
| Lebon [39] | standard | 0 | 0 | pos | | | |
| Carne [26] | + daily group sessions, used CG instead of HCG | 8 | 17 | neg | | | |

*HCG = Human chorionic gonadotropin.

†In so far as it differs from standard which is: 500 kcal day⁻¹ plus one intramuscular injection of 125 iu HCG or placebo daily over a period of 3.5 to 6 weeks.

‡a = weight-loss; b = fat-redistribution; c = hunger; d = feeling of well-being, pos = positive, neg = negative; positive and negative are results as reported by the authors in the article.

If you are not a geeky science-lover let me break down the results for you:

a. The hCG injections do not lead to greater weight loss than the diet alone

b. The hCG injections do not lead to fat distribution

c. The hCG injections do not lead to less hunger

d. The hCG injections do not lead to increased well-being

One often cited study[3-6] showed potential effect on elderly men with androgen deficiency so unless you can call yourself a part of this group, please save yourself from injecting a derivate of female urine into your muscles and stick to the diet techniques and recommendations in this book instead. You'll be better off.

## Potential side effects

Apart from being a useless supplement for fat loss here are some other reported potential adverse effects of hCG:

Arterial and venous thromboembolism, ectopic pregnancies, increased risk for multiple pregnancies, premature epiphyseal closure (stalled growth) in younger men, gynecomastia , testicular shrinkage, abdominal pain, diarrhea, water retention and hypertension just to namedrop a few. Awesome, right? Not.

*[FJ's edit: Hey now, some might actually consider things like testicular shrinkage benefits. I've always wanted smaller balls, since mine are so large!]*

*[Bojan's edit: lol, or you might have Orchitis]*

*[FJ's edit: Damn it, why must you scare me like that!? Now I'm worried. I'm emailing you a pic of my balls, please provide me with your professional opinion.]*

*[Bojan's edit: Err... I take that back, I'm sure you're just fine!]*

## Conclusions

A 500 calorie diet will lead to substantial weight loss in just about any individual. It's stupid and not sustainable for longer periods of time for the vast majority of people, but still. The effects of the hCG diet can be solely attributed to the low calorie intake and the addition to hCG injections will not lead to enhanced effects on fat loss, subjective hunger, fat distribution or what have you.

Before starting any pharmacological therapy, you always have to consider the potential wanted effects of a substance to the potential risks. In this case, we have all the potential side effects above on one side of the scale and a useless product for weight loss on the other. The choice is yours to make.

### From Sweden with love, Dr. Bojan Kostevski
*MD, personal trainer, education junkie, an overall really busy guy, with a big interest in getting folks strong and sexy.*

# Myth Busting: Separating Fact From Fiction

MYTH: **If you eat a low-fat diet, it doesn't matter how much else you eat because you won't get fat.**

Obviously, the person who made such a statement wasn't aware of my 3 laws of fat loss, and is probably walking around with an ass that is capable of eclipsing the sun while suffering from laughable hormone levels. To drop the fat off your body, the total amount of calories burnt during the day should exceed the amount of calories taken in while incorporating an intelligent exercise program.

So whether you eat a "low fat" diet, or a "low carb" diet, it doesn't matter. At the end of the day, if you took in *more* calories than you burnt off, you will eventually GAIN weight. However, it must be said that the quality of fat that you eat does matter and the basic theory goes like this: your cell walls are made up of lipids (fats) that you eat.

This can be trans fats (bad stuff) or the good stuff such as mono/polyunsaturated fats, omega-3, 6, 9 etc. When you eat the good stuff, it makes the cell walls more insulin sensitive, which will allows sugar to enter the cell easily and be used as fuel. When you eat the bad stuff, your cell walls become insulin resistive, which means sugar has a harder time entering the cell, and doesn't get burnt off. So what does your body do with this extra fuel floating around in your blood stream? It stores it as fat for later use.

**MYTH: You shouldn't lift weights often, otherwise you will get big and bulky!**

This myth is brought to you by women who watch way too many female bodybuilding shows and now PMS every time they see a loaded barbell. You do NOT get big in the gym, you get big during the recovery process along with a lifestyle that revolves around massive caloric intake.

And you know those female bodybuilders you see? They're sticking needles in their ass to increase their testosterone levels through the roof. So unless you plan on doing that, lifting weights will never make you huge. In fact, I dare you to try while on a caloric deficit.

**MYTH: If you want to lose fat you should only do aerobics, not weight lifting.**

And I heard that if you want to bake a cake, you should use a microwave, not an oven. Oh wait, does that statement sound ridiculous? Good, because that myth sounds equally as ridiculous. When it comes to helping you burn fat, cardio is basically a bowl of lame sauce[4-1] topped off with jabrony crumbs*. For a more in-depth look at cardio and how to do it effectively, read *"What About Cardio"* in Chapter 4.

**MYTH: The longer you workout in the gym, the better.**

There is an optimal, magical amount of time that you should spend on a workout whether it's in the gym or at home. This magical period of time is dependent on your personal rate of recovery, worth ethic, bad-assery and a host of other factors.

However, most people will do their bodies well by keeping their workouts under 60 minutes. Your primary focus should be to increase the density (amount of work done in the given period of time), not the duration (increasing the time spent doing half-assed physical activity).

*jabrony [jub-rony] – noun: a term used to describe something or someone as being inferior*

**MYTH: If you stop working out, your muscles will turn into fat.**

I laugh every time I hear this one because to me, it's almost as ridiculous as saying that one day your rusty pennies will turn into gold coins. It does not work like that. Fat cells are basically storage units for energy and nothing else. There is no way a muscle cell can just turn into a fat cell. This isn't the biological equivalent of Transformers, people! Although that would be rather cool... Cellulorprime vs Lipidotron!

What does happen however, is that if you stop applying resistance to your muscles, they stop adapting and eventually shrink. But if you start applying resistance again, you will be back in your groove in no time. When it comes to your muscles, use it or lose it.

**MYTH: My friend said training with weights causes you to become stiff and in-flexible.**

Does he even lift?! Probably not... because if he did, he wouldn't resort to such moronic statements. If anything, weight training can maintain, or even help increase flexibility[3-11]. The study I just cited came up with the following:

*"It was concluded that participation in a similarly structured weight training program to develop muscular strength would not impair flexibility but might increase it".*

The "stiff" feeling that people confuse with flexibility is actually the pump you get during your workouts when the blood flow has increased to the muscle group being worked. This does *not* have a negative impact on your flexibility. Which is good, because now you can keep doing your hot yoga, but please, just stay away from Zumba.

**MYTH: Women need their own special workout plan.**

I can pretty much guarantee that this statement is the result of some dumb chick obsessed with the feminist movement. So the answer is, no they don't! On a cellular level we are all the same. Women can do all the exercises than men can do, the only difference might be the amount of weight they push.

Since men naturally have more testosterone, our rate of recovery and overall strength levels are generally better, but the basic biomechanics of the exercises listed in this book do *not* need to change. So ladies, this leaves you with zero excuses. Put a bar on your back, and start squatting. Leave Hip Hop Abs and Tae Bo for the women who have an unconscious fascination with being pear shaped. If you truly want a real world idea of the results weight lifting has on the feminine physique, check out the Girls Gone Strong team.

**MYTH: When you workout you should always "feel the burn" and go to "failure"!**

Not really. It is possible to do an effective workout without 'feeling the burn'. But, the burn is there for a reason. It's the lactic acid buildup in your muscles and is an indication that you are about to reach muscular failure, which can help you know where you max intensity lies. Now, there are two schools of thought when it comes to training to failure; some say it's the best way to go, others say training to failure is stupid.

Personally, both methods of training have their uses but I tend to agree with the latter group since going to failure increases your cortisol levels (bad), reduces IGF-1 (insulin-like growth factor), reduces strength and overall power; the only benefit of training to failure is increased muscular endurance[3-12] – which makes sense since you're performing 1-2 extra repetitions per set.

**MYTH: The newest machines are better and give better results.**

No way, José! Machines have a well-deserved, shitty reputation from many top strength coaches and personal trainers who generally know what it is they are doing. Personally, I haven't bothered to touch 80% of the mechanical equipment in my gym. When friends ask me to show them how X, Y, Z machine works, my general response is "Pfft... I don't fucking know"

Apparently, because I train people I'm supposed to know how every new piece of mechanical contraption works. Well I don't have time for that crap, mainly because I'm focusing on more important things such as perfecting my Squat and Deadlift technique and breaking National Records[3-14]. Having said all of that, there is still a place for machines in your routine.

Yes, it's true... you can use pre-determined movement patterns to see results. But only if you follow the hierarchy of training. You see, your body works as an entire unit so you need to train it as such. I still don't know of a single physical task in life where you need to specifically isolate a muscle group such as you biceps. Unless you're at a gun show, I guess.

But when you train the body as a unit, there will come a time when smaller stabilizer muscle groups (such anterior and medial deltoids) will start to fatigue and give out well before the primary ones that you are trying to work (such as pectorals).

This is where machines can come into play – because they isolate a specific muscle group which can be worked to exhaustion without affecting the smaller stabilizers. Below are four categories of exercises, listed in order, that will give you maximum results in the shortest amount of time. And by results I mean muscle, strength and fat loss... which also happen to be the 3 factors of sexiness.

# The Hierarchy Of Training

## 1. Instable + Heavy Load (IH)

An IH exercise is any big compound movement which can be heavily loaded with free weights. So Deadlifts, Squats, Benchpress, PowerCleans, Overhead Press, Snatch, Overhead Squat etc. are all great examples. I refer to it as "instable" because your stabilizers will have to fire and their recruitment will play a huge role in the success of the lift. NOT because you'll be using stupid pieces of equipment such as the Bosu ball and other nonsense. The Bosu stuff is something I like to refer to as EI (Extreme Instability) exercises, which should be used only for physio/rehab purposes as far as I'm concerned.

## 2. Instable + Light Load (IL)

An IL exercise is any compound movement that cannot be loaded as heavily as an IH. So DB Bench Press, DB Pullover, Goblet Squat, Kettlebell Swings etc. Again, it's referred to as "instable" because your stabilizers will need to fire but the load that you'll be lifting will not be nearly as high as an IH exercise. If you've ever compared your maximum lift in a regular BB Bench Press to the DB Bench Press then you know exactly what I'm talking about. A guy with a solid 315lbs press will have a challenging time with 100lbs DB's in each hand.

## 3. Stable + Free Load (SF)

A SF exercise is any pre-determined movement/isolation exercise which can be loaded with free weights. So BB curls, Preacher Curls, DB Kickbacks, DB Shoulder fly etc. It is referred to as "stable" because while there is a protagonist/antagonist situation happening, the recruitment of stabilizers is very low, making the exercise itself already very stable in nature.

## 4. Stable + Load (SL)

And finally, we get to SL, which is basically anything to do with machines. So a machine preacher curl, quad extensions, ab curl nonsense, leg press, pec deck, Smith Machine bullshits etc.

There is barely any recruitment of stabilizer muscles whatsoever. The primary reason that I, or any of the other strong, logical and good looking trainers don't bother using machines is because by the time we go through IH, IL and SF exercises, we've worked hard enough to not bother with SL any nonsense.

But what do you see most idiots do? They walk into the gym and jump right on the machines faster than Charlie Sheen on a hooker. 95% of the time, if you have enough energy left to do SL exercises at the end of your routine, you probably didn't work hard enough (with minor exceptions such as the leg press). So which group of individuals make up this other 5%? Bodybuilders, and advanced trainees looking to put on muscle.

I usually prescribe a SL exercise when the primary goal is hypertrophy VIA sheer volume. Some people have muscle groups that just so fucking stubborn, that they will refuse to grow past a certain point unless you completely demolish them. Let's say that your man boobs, err... I mean chest is a particular problem area.

Here's a simple order of exercises you can follow (Sets x Reps):
5×5 BB BenchPress
4×8 DB BenchPress
3×8 Weighted Dips
3×8 DB Flys
2×15 Machine Chest Flys

If that doesn't give you a shirt-ripping chest (or give you an extra cup size for the ladies) then either you're lifting pussy weights or aren't eating enough. Point blank period. I never thought I'd be recommending machines and their use in a person's routine, but here we are.

The simple fact of the matter is that since most gyms these days are filled will machines, we need to find a decent use for them at some point in our training. As long as their presence doesn't creep into my Dumbbell, Barbell and Squat Rack area, I won't bitch too much.

**MYTH: Some legal and natural supplements work just as well as steroids without the side effects.**

Negative! There are currently no 'natural' or legal supplements that work as good as steroids. The only supplements that work better than steroids, are *other* steroids. Does this mean I am condoning steroid use? Of course not. But be aware of this little fact.

If legal compounds were as effective as steroids, why wouldn't most pro body builders use them? Do you think they like the risk of possible side effects such as man tits and a smaller ball-sack? I think not...

**MYTH: You need to do low reps & heavy weights to grow muscle and low weights and high reps to tone and change their shape.**

I hear this load of crap everywhere, specially from "trendy" trainers that have zero grasp of training knowledge and jump from one bandwagon to another, *cough* CrossFit *cough*. Listen carefully as I drop the following knowledge bomb: you CANNOT elongate or shorten the shape of your muscles by training differently (unless you resort to surgery).

Muscles will always retain their natural shape and either grow bigger and stronger or get smaller and weaker, that's it! If you want to look "toned" - lose the body fat. However, latest research[3-13] shows that low load/high rep training can be just as effective (if not more) at helping you build muscles as low load/heavy rep training. Given the data we have available, it would be wise to train both – heavy with low reps and light for high reps.

**MYTH: I heard from someone that weightlifting causes injuries!**

And I heard that same person likes running into walls head first to increase their level of intelligence.

I'm not sure from where, or from whom you heard this from but that person couldn't be more wrong if they stole an allergic kid's EpiPen for the sake of hilarity. Who you listen to is important, and since I'm important, it's probably a good idea to listen to me and accept the fact that weightlifting is downright awesome, and safe.

The only time it's "dangerous" is when you're being a dumbass and letting your ego lift the weight instead of technique, focus and a general hatred for the bar. Weightlifting is generally one of the safest things you can do. In fact, most douche-nuts think that using machines is keeping them safe when actual scientific facts reveals anything but. Let me provide you with a few direct quotes...

"Rhea (2003) suggests there is no practical difference in injury rate between using free weights or machines in healthy adults." - *Requa RK, DeAvilla LN, Garrick JG. (1993) Injuries in recreational adult fitness activities. Am J Sports Med, 21(3):461-7.*

"Injuries sustained during weightlifting training and weightlifting competition are substantially lower than injuries incurred from other sports such as football, gymnastics, or basketball." - *Stone MH (1990). Muscle conditioning and muscle injuries. Med Sci Sports Exerc. 22(4):457-462.*

"Regular participation in a broad-based training program that includes resistance training can significantly reduce sports related injuries in adolescents."- *Faigenbaum AD, Schram J (2004). Can resistance training reduce injuries in youth sports? Strength and Conditioning Journal. 26(3) 16-21.*

So basically, if weight training was any safer, it would be called Golf.

# Chapter 3 References

3-1: The term "bitch" isn't meant to be derogatory. If you haven't figured out my sense of humor by now, slap yourself for taking things too seriously.

3-2: **Increased meal frequency does not promote greater weight loss in subjects who were prescribed an 8-week equi-energetic energy-restricted diet.**

3-3: **Weight loss is greater with consumption of large morning meals and fat-free mass is preserved with large evening meals in women on a controlled weight reduction regimen.**

3-4: **The action of chorionic gonadotrophin in the obese.**

3-5: **The effect of human chorionic gonadotropin (HCG) in the treatment of obesity by means of the Simeons therapy: a criteria-based meta-analysis.**

3-6: **A Double-Blind, Placebo-Controlled, Randomized Clinical Trial of Recombinant Human Chorionic Gonadotropin on Muscle Strength and Physical Function and Activity in Older Men with Partial Age-Related Androgen Deficiency**

3-7: **Effects of resistance vs. aerobic training combined with an 800 calorie liquid diet on lean body mass and resting metabolic rate.**

3-8: **Effects of combined endurance and strength training on muscle strength, power and hypertrophy in 40-67-year-old men**

3-9: Dr.Bojan Kostevski's ILCD experiment can be read about on his site: **http://www.lift-heavy.com/ilcd-diet/**

3-10: **Effects of supplement timing and resistance exercise on skeletal muscle hypertrophy**

3-11: **Flexibility And Strength Training**

3-12: **Differential effects of strength training leading to failure versus not to failure on hormonal responses, strength, and muscle power gains**

3-13: **Low-load high volume resistance exercise stimulates muscle protein synthesis more than high-load low volume resistance exercise in young men.**

3-14: **How I Overcame Low Back Pain & Broke A National Deadlift Record**

3-15: If you have the printed version of the book, use the following link: **http://bit.ly/KZeed5**

3-16: To learn more about Eat Stop Eat, visit: **http://www.fitjerk.com/eatstopeat**

# Chapter 4: Lift Things Up, And Put Them Down (Training)

# Reps Are King

Out of all the training parameters that we have available to us, reps are king. Trainers and fitness enthusiasts argue about training concepts all the time but from my experience, knowing the number reps you *need* to perform will basically tell you everything else about your program. It will tell you what weight to use, the volume, how many sets to pull off and what results you should expect (strength, fat loss, hypertrophy etc.)

With rep manipulation, I can literally transform any workout to deliver a different result. Give me a powerlifting routine and with rep & rest tweaking I can turn it into a fat loss workout. Will it be perfectly ideal? No, but it can be done. This is a huge revelation I had because what do most people think of as the most important aspect of a workout routine? Exercises! They think the *type* of exercise will have the greatest impact on their results. Not!

Effective exercises have their place, no doubt. Just as sets, rest, tempo and load have theirs. But they are not *the* most important factor. Anyone who tells you so just hasn't been under the bar enough. Seriously. I can take some of the most biomechanically awkward exercises and by selecting the right reps (which will tell me what load to use and the total volume output etc.) deliver someone a result.

That's how powerful reps are.

So, how many should you do? For our goal, we are going to be performing exercises in the rep range of 8-15 with heavy as well as lighter loads and will cycle between these. It will provide a perfect balance of fat loss and some muscle hypertrophy[3-13]. This is what I've done for years when I wanted to cut, and the results speak for themselves.

Next, you need a little education on muscle fiber types. There are two main types of muscle fibers in our body, Slow Twitch (Type I) and fast twitch (Type II). The fast twitch fibers are broken down into two types, Type IIa and Type IIb. What the heck are these and why do you need to know this information? Because it will complete your understand of how your damn body works. So pay attention.

## Slow Twitch Muscle Fibers (Type I)

These muscle fibers are known to be oxidative. This means that they are most efficient at using oxygen as fuel to provide energy over anaerobic methods (such as using glycogen). They are called slow twitch because they take longer to fire than other fibers but on the flip side, they can function for hours before becoming fatigued. If you are a long distance runner/marathoner then your body is probably made up of these fibers.

## Fast Twitch Muscle Fibers (Type IIa)

These are known as the intermediate fibers because of their well rounded ability to use aerobic (oxygen) and anaerobic (glycogen) methods of producing energy. Think of them as the Jack-of-all-trade type of muscle fiber. But, although they can use oxygen for energy, they do not last as long as Type I fibers. Individuals into body building, martial arts, sprinting or any other high energy sport should consider focusing on these muscle fibers.

## Fast Twitch Muscle Fibers (Type IIb)

These are the classic fast-twitch fibers which most people have in mind. Think of them as a powerful yet relatively short-lived turbo boost. This is because they rely completely on glycogen stores for energy and once these stores are depleted, they undergo exhaustion. Type II fibers are also the thickest and therefore have the highest potential for growth.

So, how do you know you have fast twitch or slow twitch muscles? Easy, just look at your past experiences. One huge fallacy that fitness "gurus" and trainers are preaching is the fact that if you are slow twitch, then you'll always be slow twitch. This is a load of faggotry. If muscles can adapt to stress and then grow, why can't they adapt to the rate at which they fire? Well the good news is that they can, and they do.

If you've done tons and tons of low intensity cardio and sissy ass weights in the past, then chances are that you are comprised mainly of slow twitch fibers, while others are just born slow twitch. And if you were a track athlete and used to explosive bouts of running, jumping etc., chances are that you're muscles are mainly fast-twitch.

So to change things around, you will have to change your training. Your muscles will adapt to whatever you do. Start throwing in some explosiveness during the concentric phase of every lift and make sure the load is 70-80% of your 1 rep maximum and you'll be fast twitching your way to sexy land.

# Sets

So what are sets? A set is a group that includes a specific number of reps done consecutively. So if you do 8 reps and stop, you just completed one set. In the first version of Flawless Fitness, I stated that that sets are inversely proportional to the number of reps you do, and here is the fancy custom chart I made along with the explanation...

| Number of Reps | | |
|---|---|---|
| 1 2 3    4 5 6 7 9    10    12 15 20 | | |
| High | Medium | Low |
| (10 - 6) | (5 – 3) | (3 - 1) |
| Number of Sets | | |

Now after you look at that, I am sure you are thinking either one of two things:
"Forget sets, what was his beer count when he made that up?!"
"Hmm... that sort of makes sense to me!"

If you fall into category #2, you may skip the next two paragraphs. If however you fall into category #1, or are just plain curious, let me explain. Yes the numbers seem vague, partially missing, and all over the place, but that's because I tried to make this as accurate as possible.

The thing is, you cannot be PERFECT with this. There is no 100% clear answer and it's not written in stone because everyone is different. This table is as close as it gets to perfection, in my jerkacious opinion. You can say otherwise, but you'd probably be wrong.

So how do you use it? Let's say you decided to do about 15 reps. Using my "Set spectrum of awesomeness" you now fall into the 'low' end. So should you do 1, 2 or 3 sets? Usually one set is not the greatest idea for 15 reps so I would say 2 sets. Ok, how about 9 reps? Well that almost falls under the number three, so 3 sets. See... it's not that hard.

## A New Way Of Looking At Sets

Everything I stated above still holds true, but when it comes to fat loss, I found that there is a method that is even more ass kicking – I call it *sets in relation to muscle size*. See, if you do 10 reps for 3 sets for your biceps, you'll probably trigger a decent amount of growth and will work them to exhaustion (assuming you used a challenging enough weight). I really don't see why you'd need to do anymore work.

But if you use the exact same parameters for your chest, then there is no way you'll have challenged your pectorals to their limits. Compared to the biceps, the chest is a huge muscle group, which means it can handle more work and therefore it needs a bigger trashing; so basically, you need more sets. Something in the rage of 5-7 would be ideal.

And for the growth monsters out there who want to get a bigger chest, swapping between the two methods above – the inverse relationship between sets/reps and set range in relation to muscle size will give you tits so big you'll need a bra. No joke. For women... just know that you'll burn lots and lots of calories.

# Tempo

Tempo refers to the speed of your lift. Most people have no clue what tempo is and therefore every lift they perform is done at the same speed. As a result, their lifts stagnate. Just as how your body will get used to a certain routine, so too will it get used to a certain tempo - so it makes sense that we change this around once in a while.

Now that you know the basic definition of tempo, you need to know how to read it and apply it. Usually, it's expressed in three digits like so → 311. This used to confuse me at first, so for the sake of better understanding I'll write tempo as 3-1-1 in this section. Once you know what each number means though, it won't matter, you'll be able to read tempo easily.

Let's use 3-1-1 to explain:

**First # (3):** This number represents the eccentric part of an exercise (where your muscles elongate). For example, if you are doing squats with a tempo of 3-1-1, it should take you 3 seconds to sink down from a standing position. Or for a bench press, it should take you 3 seconds to lower the bar towards your chest.

**Second #(1):** This number represents the amount of time you should stay in an isometric position. In this case, the number is 1. So again, if you are doing squats, after you sink down you will hold that position for 1 second. Or for a bench press, you will keep the bar an inch above your chest for 1 second.

**Third #(1):** This number represents the concentric phase (when your muscles contract) of an exercise. So for the squats, you would stand up within one second, and for the bench press, you would press the bar upwards for a 1 second count. Sometimes this # can be expressed as an "X" which means as fast as humanly possible... or in other words, use explosive power.

## What Tempo Should You Use?

There have been a crap load of studies done that measure the specific performance of an athlete based on the tempo they use during training; so you would think that the subject of tempo selection for an exercise would be conclusive. But many strength coaches and fitness experts tend to have conflicting opinions when it comes to tempo... and judging by the online arguments that still pop up weekly, it seems that these arguments will continue on for decades to come. Oh think of the children!

So what I'm going to do is try and explain *why* this tempo war is happening and my take on it. I'm not going to make a bold statement and say that my way is the only way, but it's been tested by me in my little "inner" circle enough times that I believe it will give you the results you want in the shortest amount of time possible.

Charles Staley (creator of Escalating Density Training) believes that the human body is designed for accelerative and ballistic type of stress (think throwing a baseball, jumping etc.) and is therefore a supporter of fast and explosive tempo. But coaches such as Charles Poliquin seem to favor slower tempos around the 3-5 second rage for the eccentric phase of the lift (usually speaking).

But I've adopted a hybrid approach from Christian Thibaudeau and it has given me the best results. There is no guess work when it comes to eccentric training - it has shown to be superior when it comes to maximizing muscle hypertrophy and strength *[Higby et al. 1996, Hortobagyi et al. 1996, Grabiner and Owings 2002, Linnamo et al. 2002, Martin et al. 1995]*

But the strength and size gains that come from eccentric training need to be functional, and for that to happen you need to make sure the concentric part of any lift is done as explosively as possible. However, we need to remember that we aren't purely after strength and size... we want to get as ripped as possible; therefore every time we do work, we need to undergo maximum calorie burnage!

The easiest way to do this is to increase your time under tension. One rep of a squat that takes 8 seconds to complete will burn more calories than a squat that you complete in 3 seconds (assuming the load remains the same). But I also don't want you to become slow and have the athletic ability of a couch rider. So my suggestion is to alternate.

Use a tempo of **3-0-X** for 4 weeks, then swap it out for **4-1-4**. We won't bother with eccentric tempos around the 1-2 second range since that is what most people do anyways and it's what your body is probably used to if you've trained before... and you don't want to look like *most* people now do you? I sure as hell hope not.

**Quick Word On Explosive Tempo ("X")**

A few people always get confused by the letter "X" when written in tempo format and I need to make sure that there are no confusions on your part. Your understanding of this should be absolutely clear. Applying *your* maximal force to a load and visually seeing that load move at an explosive rate are two completely different things. We want the former, not the latter. Moving 5lbs as fast as possible is considered an explosive movement, but it won't get you the results you seek.

Let's say you are about to bench press 90% of your one rep max (1RM) for a given tempo. So you lower the bar for a count of three, hold it for a second, then *try* and explosively push that bar away from you as fast as possible. To a bystander however, it might look like the concentric portion of the lift was actually 4 seconds, not "X". So what should you write down? 314 or 31X?

If you said 31X then pat yourself on the back, you now understand explosive tempo. If you didn't, then question your true IQ and re-read this entire section. The point of explosive tempo is to *try* and overcome the resistance as fast as *you* possibly can, but it doesn't mean you'll be able to. Especially when you are lifting some heavy ass shit.

But the point is that your neural drive is being optimized and therefore you will reap the benefits. When powerlifters deadlift 800lbs, they are actually performing a concentric tempo of "X" even though it can take them 5 seconds to hit lockout from the point of liftoff.

# Load (Weight Used)

So now that you know how many times you should lift weights and with what speed, it's time to talk about how much weight you should load up on the bar before attempting a brutal battle with gravity. There are two ways to go about it. One way is to find your 1RM, which is the amount of weight you can lift for a maximum of one rep, then select a percentage of that. Or, you can adjust and eyeball your weight on the fly by follow my advice that "reps are king".

When I'm aiming for fat loss, I follow the latter method and when I'm doing any type of strength or hypertrophy training, I like to get more scientific and play around with percentages of my 1RM.

Since the goal of this book is to get you lean and mean, I'll say that you should listen to your body and test out the necessary load you can lift for your prescribed number of reps. A few things to keep in mind when it comes to the amount of load on the bar:

Leave your ego behind (this is more for the bros). There is an obvious inverse relationship between the number of reps you can do and the amount of weight you can lift. The higher the reps, the lighter you'll have to lift. Don't be a hero... no one gives a flying squirrel dump that you can do more reps than the guy beside you. You do what *you* need to do, and do it safely.

Even though we won't really be using percentages of 1RM, I would still like you to figure out your 1RM for the following four exercises: Benchpress, Deadlift, Squat & Overhead Press to see where your strength levels are at. Do it once or twice a month. Oh, and this doesn't mean using fancy formulas, rep max calculators and all that other bullshit.

The only true way to find your 1RM is to do the lifts.

The reason I don't like formulas is because there are too many variables to consider in the real world. Some people will have longer arms; therefore their deadlift ability will be well beyond what a formula can predict, while another person might be tall and have extremely long legs, making squatting a challenge etc. So get a spotter, do your one rep maxes, and record them.

**The 2.5lbs plate is your best friend**.

Besides the bar itself, there is no other "weight" that I use more in the gym than the 2.5's. Your job is to always progress from one workout to the next. If that is too soon, then try progressing every other workout. If you are putting in a maximal amount of effort, there is no reason you shouldn't be able to throw on 2.5lbs every few sessions.

This type of progress is also known as "progressive overload". I'm not sure why this technique is only used for strength training, because it acts as rocket fuel when applied to any fat loss program.

# Rest – How Much?

One of the most confusing aspects of training, at least for me, was knowing how much I should rest. There were just too many things to think about. The nervous system needs 36-48 hours to recover, then you also have muscle size to consider - so if I worked legs then I'd probably need to chill out for a longer period of time then when I worked my arms. Then we have supplements which can help reduce recovery time etc. Throw all these variables into a mix and you're left with one confusing scenario.

But when you just want to get lean as hell, the bottom line is that you need to be burning calories and getting your metabolic rate up as often as possible. Adding cardio is a good way to do this without burning yourself out too much, but I like to avoid useless running. I want to get ripped in the most efficient way possible – with the least amount of expended effort in the shortest amount of time.

That leaves me with one option (if you haven't noticed by now) which is weight training. (**Note:** Cardio will be covered later on, so for all you running lovers, don't get your aerodynamic spandexes in a bunch.)

Since I like to move away from complexity and towards simplicity, I've come to the conclusion that a 24hour period, augmented with some supplementation is sufficient when trying to get lean. So if you have a 4day/week plan, then a training schedule on Monday, Wednesday, Friday, Sunday works. Now you might be thinking, "but FJ, the day after Sunday is Monday, so that means I'll get no rest!", to which I say "good eye, young grasshoppa!"

Your week2 will start on Tuesday and end on a Monday. Week3 will start on Wednesday and end on Tuesday. By the time you're done any 4 week plan, you'll have finished on a Wednesday assuming you started off on a Monday.

Most think that just because you started your workout plan at the beginning of our traditional work week (Monday) that you need to end on a Sunday every time. Uh... no! Your workout days will follow a strict schedule regardless of what "day" it happens to land on.

A new week starts only when you've finished a previous "workout week", and a new workout session only starts after a twenty-four hour period. No exceptions. (See the table below in case a massively confused look has appeared on your face right now...)

## A 4 Week Workout Plan With 24hr Rest Periods

| Workout Week | Workout Day | Workout Day | Workout Day | Workout Day |
|---|---|---|---|---|
| Week 1 | Day1 (Mon) | Day2 (Wed) | Day3 (Fri) | Day4 (Sun) |
| Week 2 | Day5 (Tue) | Day6 (Thurs) | Day7 (Sat) | Day8 (Mon) |
| Week 3 | Day9 (Wed) | Day10 (Fri) | Day11 (Sun) | Day12 (Tue) |
| Week 4 | Day13 (Thurs) | Day14 (Sat) | Day15 (Mon) | Day16 (Wed) |

This would be an ideal setup for the ordinary person. However, if you want to be extra-ordinary, then you'll have to train daily. Or god forbid, multiple times per day. What's that I hear you say? Overtraining? More like over-pussyfication. I realize that the "train daily" statement goes against everything anyone has ever told you, but if you keep doing what "they" are telling you, you'll end up just as fat, as "they" are.

The simple fact of the matter is that the human body can withstand enormous amounts of volume when it comes to training. And while the initial week will suck, you will eventually get used to the high volume work load and adapt rather quickly. As such, results will come quickly as well.

Honestly, if the 300lbs+ warpigs in *The Biggest Loser* TV show can manage to train 8 hours *per day*, I think you can manage a daily one-hour workout schedule without worrying about "overtraining". So how exactly do you manage rest and recovery with a higher than average training volume? You make sure what you eat is spot-on.

And enlist the help of supplementation, which we'll get to in chapter 5. Also, ensure that if you are training daily, your workouts are under an hour long. Aim for intensity and density – lots of heavy work done in a short amount of time.

# Variation

This principal is so stupidly simple, I can't seem to recall why I dedicated an entire section to it. Oh wait, now I remember why – to illustrate that it's important as hell! So, variation... the idea is very basic: **Change up your workout routine every 6-8weeks, or sooner if you're horrendously bored to tears.** The reasoning behind it is that your body is extremely good at adapting to stress. After 6 weeks, I found that the results produced by most routines started to dip.

I've also experimented by changing things up every 4 weeks, and seems to work well also. I also know guys that change up their workouts every week, which is not only detrimental to progress, but also highly un-necessary. If it entices you though, or if you suffer from an extreme case of STEED (Short Term Exercise Excitement Disorder), then weekly changes is something you might want to try, but not daily.

The general rule is this – if you're beginner, intermediate or under the watchful eye of a coach, changing up your routine too frequently is a bad idea. If however, you've been 'around the block' and just want to try shit out, changes can be made more frequently and on the fly because you'll know exactly what your body can, or cannot handle on the given day.

For example, when it comes to strength training, I've stopped with the linear progressive overload model because I cannot gain strength in that fashion anymore. My strength gains now resemble a wave and so I adapt as such. And that's all you need to know on variation.

Well that was a short... talk about getting right to the point. Since I had all this empty space and didn't know what to do with it, I figured I'd throw in a few quotes I find amusing...

*These days many people get their exercise jumping to conclusions, flying off the handle, dodging responsibilities, bending the rules, running down everything, circulating rumors, passing the buck, stirring up trouble, shooting the bull, digging up dirt, slinging mud, throwing their weight around, beating the system, and pushing their luck.*

----

*"If you're so into fitness and sex, why don't you take a f\*\*king hike!"*
(Found on a T-Shirt)

----

*"At my gym they have free weights, so I took them." -- Steve Smith*

----

*"If swimming is so good for your figure, explain whales to me!" - Unknown*

----

*I decided to take an aerobics class. I bent, twisted, gyrated and jumped up and down for an hour. But, by the time I got my leotards on, the class was over. -Unknown*

----

*Exercise must be good for you. My wife's tongue has never been sick a day in her life. -Unknown*

----

*Is there a rule that the older you are in the locker room at the gym, the more naked you have to be? – Kyle Cease*

----

*God must love calories since he made so many! -Unknown*

----

*"The word aerobics comes from two Greek words: aero, meaning "ability to," and bics, meaning "withstand tremendous boredom" ~ Dave Barry*

# On Bodyweight Training

If it wasn't clear enough already, I'm going to do the unthinkable and repeat myself – I think getting a gym membership is one of the best investments you can make. However, don't let anyone preach to you that getting in great shape with bodyweight training is impossible... because it isn't. It just might take a bit longer.

The biggest hurdle when doing bodyweight training is the ability to scale your resistance level. If you are really out of shape, then your own bodyweight becomes something that is un-manageable and if you've been working out for a long time, then applying the required amount of stress to your muscles becomes a challenging task.

But being involved with gymnastics, bodyweight training is pretty much all we do, and I'm going to share some kick ass bodyweight exercises that you can do and some clever methods to enhance their resistance levels. You might have heard of some of these exercises while others might be a bit alien to you, but the only thing you need to know is that they work, and they work really well.

To this day, I still throw in bodyweight training into my normal routines because while pushing heavy weights is one thing, knowing how to push your own weight around is vitally important. Specially for those that are involved in sports.

The first thing I'm going to talk about, are ways to enhance your bodyweight exercises in case they are a bit too easy for you. Here's the list...

**Angle Manipulation:** Are pushups too easy? Try doing them by having your feet up on an incline so your body makes a 45degreen angle with the floor. Still too easy? Try handstand pushups; where you'll be perpendicular to the floor. Are normal sit-ups dragging you down lame street? Try doing them off the end of a bench where you can have a greater range of motion and go below your seated level.

If a bodyweight exercise ever becomes easy, the first thing you should ask yourself is "Is there a way I can change the angle to increase resistance?"

**Increase Tempo:** At a normal pace, I can probably bang out about 50 pushups without much trouble. However, change the tempo to something like 412 and now all of a sudden that number drops to 20. Even if the resistance level is light (as is the case with bodyweight training), you can increase the effectiveness by increasing your time under tension. Here is an athlete doing a 2 minute chin-up! Video Link: **http://www.youtube.com/watch?v=_23cl5n8NaQ** If you were to write out the tempo, that would be 60-0-60. Intense? Oh, you bet it is.

**Bodyweights:** This method costs a bit of cash but is quite worth it in my opinion because bodyweights can not only benefit your usual exercises, but can help you increase performance in almost any other sport. Things like ankle weights, wrist weights (you can use ankle weights on your hands as well) and heavy torso vests can go a long way in improving your workouts.

If you are into combat sports, they become even more invaluable. If you don't have some cash on the side to spend, a very inexpensive option is the backpack. Load it up with some frozen peas, big cans of soup and 2L bottle of water, and you can easily add like 30lbs on your back. Now try doing pushups and jumping squats – you can hate me later.

**Multiply:** Take all those of the above-mentioned modifications and apply them together. Imagine doing a handstand pushup with a 31X tempo with 5lbs ankle weights and a 30lbs chest vest. It will turn weak boys into men and sissy girls into feisty ladies. Rawr.

So those are some of the best ways you can enhance your bodyweight exercises. Now it's time to discuss the exercises themselves.

Below, I've compiled a list of exercises that I believe are some of the best. If there are exercises on that list that are too advanced for you at the moment, try an alternative.

For example: If you can't do a muscle up, perform pull-ups and dips separately. If you have trouble finding alternatives, or if any of these exercises confuse you, then Google them or shoot me an email here: **flawlessfitness.ebook@gmail.com.** Alternatively, hit up my YouTube channel because as time passes, I will be throwing up tutorials/demos on all the exercises listed in this book. You can do so here: **http://www.youtube.com/user/fitjerk**

| Pushup (Normal/Wide/1Hand) | Squat Jumps | Pistol Squats |
|---|---|---|
| Squats (Normal or Hindu) | Dive Bombers | Mountain Climbers |
| Dips/Chair Dips | Towel Pullups | Jumping Lunges |
| Pullups | Muscle Ups | Reverse Grip Pushups |
| Chinups | Inch Worm | Hill Sprints |
| Handstands | Spiderman Walk | Penguin Walk (on P.Bars) |
| Handstand Pushup | Tuck Jumps | Calf Raises |
| Plank | Bridge (Tabletop if beginner) | Hyperextensions |
| Hamstring Raises | Flagpole | Stair Climbs |

And yes I know what you're probably saying to yourself, "why aren't all these exercises explained with pretty pictures surrounded by boxes of densely worded text that put me to sleep?!", and the answer is because I wanted to keep the size of this book as lean as possible.

If I were to take every exercise mentioned in this book and try to explain them all, then the page count would easily shoot past 400 – but on the bright side, it would make a great dumbbell replacement.

While that would no doubt be handy, the massive amount of embedded pictures would really bloat up the .pdf or .epub file size and would make downloading a complete nightmare for those that have slow connections, but insist on living in the digital age.

So due to my inability to include massive tutorials, I've come up with an "as needed" solution for those of you with the digital pro version of this book. Included as per your free consultation, if you want to make sure your exercise technique is on point you can send me a video clip of you doing a particular exercise to the exclusive email address, and I'll send you feedback within 24-48 hours depending how funny looking your form is. Be sure to attach the digital receipt for proof of purchase. And remember these two key rules:

**Make sure the video is no longer than 60 seconds (1) and that the quality isn't horrible(2).** I should be able to see your entire body and make out your limbs, at the minimum. Your face doesn't matter. Wear a scream mask for all I care. The format you shoot in doesn't really matter either... I can pretty much find a way to play and/or convert any format but I don't want your home made version of TaeBo. Just be quick and to the point.

# The Best Fat-Loss Exercises

Exercise selection is going to play a huge role in how quickly you see results. If you choose to ignore my recommendations below, start doing your own thing, or do exercises your friends told you about, then don't complain when you suffer from second hand suck, and ask me *why* it's taking forever to see results. Also, don't try and substitute, replace or god forbid, modify the exercises listed below.

They work really well just as they are, and have stood the test of time. (Note: The exercises on the next page are exclusively based on using equipment since bodyweight exercises were already covered in the previous section.)

As time passes, I will be throwing up a tutorial for each one of these exercises on my YouTube channel. Hit up the link below...

**http://www.youtube.com/user/fitjerk/videos**

**BB = Barbell**
**DB = Dumbbell**
**KB = Kettle bell**

| **Full Body** | **Upper Body Dominant** |
|---|---|
| BB Lunge Press | BB Bench Press (flat/incline) |
| BB Overhead Squat | BB Pendlay Rows (Straight or |
| BB Deadlifts (Snatch Grip or | W-bar) |
| Sumo) | BB High Pulls |
| BB PowerClean | BB Close Grip Bench |
| DB Farmer Walks | BB Overhead Press (standing |
| DB Figure 8 Walks | military or push press) |
| Suitcase Deadlifts | Chinups/Pullups (Normal or |
| KB Swings | weighted) |
| | Dips (Normal or weighted) |
| **Lower Body Dominant** | Weighted Clapping Pullups |
| BB Squat (Normal, Front or | Seated Rows |
| Zercher) | DB Pullovers |
| Kneeling Jump Squat | DB Chest Flys |
| DB Lunges | DB Bench Press |
| DB Calf Raises | Standing DB Shoulder Press |
| BB Step Ups | BB Goodmornings |
| Quad Extensions | Seated DB Clean & Press |
| Hamstring Curls (or Glue- | |
| Ham Raises) | |
| Duck Leg Press | |
| Squat Jumps | |
| BB Side Lunges | |
| DB Goblet Squat | |

# What About Cardio?

Also known as aerobics... or in my world, "running for no apparent reason". While I know that it's completely possible to strip the fat off your ass without even a blip of cardio, I won't ignore this type of training just because I happen to dislike it. Truth is that there are people out there who actually *like* running, and to them I say, "good for you... crazy weirdo." But hey, to each their own. For the time being let's forget about whether you like to do it or not, and get down to the facts.

First of all, traditional cardio by itself isn't terribly effective after an initial period of 4-6 weeks for most people. In fact, doing long-term cardio is an easy way to completely waste your time while achieving pathetically modest results at best, and this has been well documented[4-1]. Let me quote the conclusion which the researchers came up with during one study:

*"Moderate-intensity aerobic exercise programs of 6-12 months induce a modest reduction in weight and waist circumference in overweight and obese populations. Our results show that **isolated aerobic exercise is not an effective weight loss therapy** in these patients. Isolated aerobic exercise provides modest benefits to blood pressure and lipid levels and may be an effective weight loss therapy in conjunction with diets."*

Do you want a "modest" result? Is that why you bought this book? I think not. So while general, long duration cardio sucks, the right kind of cardio *can* improve results when you take advantage of the following three factors:

- In conjunction with a resistance training program.
- The initial 4-6 week window.
- Performing it at the right intensities.

Let's talk about that first factor, because most people are just plain doing it wrong, and I want you to start doing shit right. Here's what "most people" do: They hit the gym, lift a bunch of light-ass weights, pound the silly machines then hop on a treadmill for another hour. What a waste of life. Now, will they be burning calories? Yes, but they'll also be doing their resistance training program an injustice.

The primary goal should be to burn maximum number of calories, without sacrificing the loss of muscle tissue. People can lose all the weight they want, but they'll look just as soft as they used to if they don't put on some muscle. And why in the world would you want to look all soft and "normal" when you can look ripped and awesome? It makes no sense to me. Anyways, back to the question at hand - Why is it an injustice if you do cardio right after a weightlifting session?

To answer this question we first have to look at an example. Have you ever noticed how most Ironman marathon runners look skinny and sometimes frail? They are no doubt very athletic and are the complete opposite of what most would consider "obese". Also, distance wise they could probably out-run me any day of the week... but ask them to throw 400+ pounds on a bar then pull it. It won't happen. And even if they tried, I guarantee their wall-flower frame will snap in half.

The bottom line is that their bodies are trained for efficiency, not power – since that's the type of training they are basically doing. So when you run around like a hamster all day long, you are training your body to mimic the engine of a Toyota Prius – small, unexciting, weak, and thus resulting in using less fuel (calories) over a longer period of time.

But we can't afford to be Priuses. We need to be the resource hogging, baby seal killing, oil company supporting, extremely fast revving, race bred Ferraris. What are Ferrari's good at? Speed, power and performance. Period.

What do they do when they idle? Eat up a shit load of fuel. What happens when you look at its V8 engine under the hood? You get excited, and your Southern bits start to tingle... at least if you're man it does. Women... just imagine a high end purse from Coach. Or maybe a shiny new pair of Jimmy Choo's.

Again, the point is that your body will adapt to the way in which you train. So when you resistance train, you're training your muscles to get bigger, become stronger, to use their stored glycogen for fuel, and become more metabolically active. The problem occurs when you try and do both. While incredibly adaptive, your body just cannot be both a Prius and a Ferrari. You can't have 590 horsepower but also expect to get 80 miles to the gallon. You need to pick one. At this point, I'll assume you've smartened up and have chosen to be the red Italian beast. Zoom-Zoom! Oh wait, that's a Mazda. Whatever.

So let's talk about how I actually do cardio without becoming a Prius. "Very quickly & infrequently", is the short and simple answer. At this point, I'll do cardio about once or twice a week and it will consist of hill sprints, jump rope, interval running, Prowler pushing, 40 yard dashes or some mangled permutation of these hideously taxing activities. On other days, I might throw in some low intensity stuff like the stationary bike (or a bike ride for real, you know, like going *outside*). However, all of this is never combined with any of my weightlifting workouts. This assures that I don't have to worry about the 4-6 week tapering effect, and since the intensity is brutal, it always works. Let's take an example of a routine I did recently...

### FitJerk's Lung Busting Cardio Routine

| Activity | Rest | Duration (s) | Sets | Intensity |
|---|---|---|---|---|
| A1 - Jump Rope | 45 | 60 | 3 | High |
| A2 - Jogging | - | 180 | - | Low |
| B1 - Hill Sprints | 60 | N/A | 4 | High |
| B2 - Jogging | - | 180 | - | Low |

So what exactly am I doing here? Well the first thing you need to know is that A1, A2, B1 and B2 are supersets. For those that have never seen something like this before, you would do A1, immediately followed by A2 then rest for 45 seconds. This would be considered one super set, and then you would repeat this 2 more times making a total of 3 sets as written. After all three, you would move on to B1 and B2 and rest for 60 seconds between each super set and do it a total of four times. Pretty straight forward stuff.

Next is the duration, which is again pretty standard. For the jump rope, you whip that sucker around as fast as you can for one minute. The only reason hill sprints has no duration is because no two hills are obviously the same. My suggestion is to find the biggest hill you can with the most absurd incline imaginable. Then try and get to the top as if a piece of chocolate cake awaits your arrival. Of course, there will be no cake, only a pool of your own sweat. The cake is a lie.

That pretty much covers it. As you begin to progress in your cardio journey, you can substitute the exercises, increase the number of sets or even add in more super sets. However, if you already have an ass busting weightlifting routine for the week, doing more than 4 super sets isn't necessary unless you're an MMA fighter and your level of conditioning is of prime importance. Or if you just like variety along with destroying yourself... then by all means, go for it.

**Substitutions:**

While there isn't a substitution for the jump rope or the 40 yard dash, you can substitute hill sprints with a treadmill that has the ability to incline and a huge tire attached to some TRX bands for the Prowler. The way it works is simple - loop a chain around the rim of the tire and attach your TRX bands to the chain. Now turn around, facing away from the tire, and hold the TRX bands in front of you (as if you just finished a rep of a cable chest press) and start walking.

It puts you in that similar, disgusting, lactic-acid inducing, low angle position as pushing the Prowler... but this time the load is behind you instead of in front. It's not as good as the Prowler, but it takes more stabilization and is as close as you can get. The point is to start dragging a huge amount of weight from a dead stop over a particular distance. If you're in average shape, you'll most probably hate doing this, but will be astonished at the results.

And to be honest, *the stuff you hate doing the most, is the stuff you need to do the most* - this piece of wisdom comes from personal experience, straight up. Follow it, and it will serve you well for the rest of your life.

# Chapter 4 References

4-1: **Isolated aerobic exercise and weight loss: a systematic review and meta-analysis of randomized controlled trials**
4-2: **Charles Poliquin on CrossFit**

# Chapter 5: Every Hero Needs A Sidekick (Supplements)

# Supplementing Supplements With Reality Pills

Drinking vitamin mixtures to replace breakfast, popping diet pills for lunch and eating protein bars for dinner are just a few examples of really the stupid shit that I've seen people do with supplements. The problem seems to be one of two things: either the general population has forgotten the English definition, or assumes that you can completely replace regular whole foods with packaged absurdity.

**Supplementation ≠ substitution.** So if you happen to come across a person that has lost their way, let me re-define the term, which you can regurgitate into their face as and when you please...

*Supplements [sup-ple-ments] –noun,*
*1. A substance added to diet or lifestyle to make up for a deficiency, or extend or strengthen a plan that is already in place and working.*
***Example:*** *"John, being the smart chap that he is, used a whey protein shake to supplement his well balanced dinner in order to meet his nutritional requirements set by his trainer."*

While outright substitution of food is one problem, another seems to be the magic solution hoopla that people keep falling for. Granted, the (clever) marketing departments of the supplement companies are partially to blame, but in the end it is your job to decide what you will end up swallowing as the truth. No pun intended. As you recall from my first law of fat loss; you cannot lose fat if you consume *more* crap from supplement companies.

## The Supplement Reward Principal

I'm going to let you in on a phenomenon I've been noticing over the years. At first, I figured it was just me, but as I started talking to other smart individuals, it seems my suspicions maybe correct.

Just as the "rich get richer", some supplements work better as the "lean get leaner." What this means is that if you're walking around at 20% body fat and start taking supplements that contain stimulants and recovery agents, you won't notice the results as much as someone who walks around at single digit body fat levels.

Physiologically the reasoning is quite simple – leaner individuals generally have better blood flow, less stress, better hormonal balance etc., and thus benefit from the extra help from the supplements at a faster, more noticeable rate. Getting back to my car analogies; what happens if you put 97 octane fuel in your Toyota Corolla? Not much. You might get *slightly* better mileage and *slightly* smoother engine response but beyond that, it's a waste of cash. However, what happens when you put such a potent liquid inside a Lamborghini? A *massive* boost in power, torque and throttle response. So if you want to get the most bang for your buck out of the supplements you buy, lose the fat!

Yeah I know, it's not fair... but that's life. As Mr.Ludacris (one of my favorite rappers) once said, "It's not the hand that you're dealt, it's how you're playing your cards, boy!"[5-1]

**Note:** *If you would like to see my highly informative and equally hilarious supplement flowchart (has over 1000 facebook shares!) click the following* link:
*http://flawlessfitnessbook.com/supplement_flowchart.html*

**The "Bro It Totally Works" Effect (Placebo)**

There resides an interesting article over at WIRED on how Placebos are getting stronger[5-2] in humans, resulting in drug companies having to ditch the testing and production of new drugs because they usually fair no better than a lame ol' sugar pill. In fact, at times the sugar pill outperforms the drug being tested. How incredibly insane is that?

Personally I'm glad, as this will result in less drugs out in the market. How? Because if you want to get a drug approved by the FDA, there needs to be proof that it works better than its placebo counterpart. This just goes to show the substantial capacity for the human body to evolve and actually heal itself without the use of external chemical substances. Here's a quote from the article, *"The fact that an increasing number of medications are unable to beat sugar pills has thrown the industry into crisis. The stakes could hardly be higher. In today's economy, the fate of a long-established company can hang on the outcome of a handful of tests."*

Love it.

Then I got thinking... is this all sunshine and lollipops? Nope, because where there is progress, there is also an exploit for opportunity. For one, drug companies are clearly upset by this placebo shit-show and what it seems to be doing to their profit margins. Therefore, they are looking into producing drugs that will *negate* the effects of placebo in patients in the first place - which I think is messed up and quite infuriating, to be honest.

But what else can you expect from these money hungry whores in disguise, who must constantly drop to their knees in order to please their shareholders? The good news is that doctors are now combining the power of placebo with normal drugs in the best interest of the patient: *"Nearly half of the doctors polled in a 2007 survey in Chicago admitted to prescribing medications they knew were ineffective for a patient's condition—or prescribing effective drugs in doses too low to produce actual benefit—in order to provoke a placebo response."*

It seems there exists a ray of hope. But then we have the supplement companies. I mean seriously, if I was the CEO of one, and I read the article from *Wired*... my entrepreneurial business mind would go off like the Spidey sense, and I'd pump out even more useless powders backed by out-of-this-world marketing claims. Why? Because as absurd as it sounds, on some level it might actually work! Customers might actually start to "feel" the benefits of the useless powders, even though it's just the evolution of the all mighty placebo effect. And hey, the doctors are doing it.

This brings me to the point I'm trying to make - while I'm clearly joking around, this type of shenanigans is actually going on inside the supplement industry, and you need to ensure the ingredients you're paying money for actually work – this is the primary reason I decided to be sponsored under AAEFX.

There is a reason 99.9% of supplements *don't* go through a double-blind placebo controlled test before being released on the market... it's just not required. This is how you and I get bombarded with completely worthless products that end up being scams such as: acai berry, resveratrol, L-Arginine (the main ingredient in "pump" products) etc.

But have you ever bothered to look beyond the label claims? If not, you should be reading my supplement reviews[5-25] (now that's what I call a smooth plug).

# Supplements That Work!

I was going write up a bunch of different lists; supplements that don't work, might work and ones that do work... but then I realized such a task in itself was too much work. So instead, I trimmed the fat, saved my fingers from tedious hours of flexion/extension and can now reveal a list of stuff that works! If it's not on the list, don't bother with it. If you feel that a certain supplement deserves to be included, hit me an email. If it's legit, I'll consider its inclusion in future editions of the book, of which there shall be many so I can keep this from becoming obsolete.

### Multivitamin

Cheap, effective and can take care of any holes in your diet plan. A multivitamin is the shotgun in your fat loss tool box that fires sticky tack and duct tape. If you follow the nutritional guidelines and food list I've provided, then you probably won't need it. But it's better to be safe than sorry.

I don't care what you buy nor from who you buy. Indulge your inner child and buy the gummy multivitamins like I do at times. You can get your candy fix and daily micronutrients all in one go, so why wouldn't you?

## Protein (Whey)

You already know what protein is from Chapter 2, so I won't spend much time going over the basics. All you need to know about whey is that it's a liquid by-product of cheese production, the fastest absorbing out of all other protein supplements, and contains about 20-25% BCAA's (Branched Chain Amino Acids). Whey is the reason I think people who pay for and take pure BCAA's are complete doorknobs.

There is no need! It's already in whey protein which happens to be relatively inexpensive, and if you buy the right formula and/or flavor, it can be a delicious treat to boot. Pure BCAA's on the other hand, usually aren't (with the exception of Xtend™ which tastes decent). I'm all about bang for your buck.

There are a bunch of different types of whey proteins (Whey isolate, whey concentrate, whey hydrolysate etc.) and each have their own little benefit. Isolate yields the most amount of protein per scoop and is so pure, those that are lactose intolerant shouldn't have any problems taking it (I'd still double check with your doctor).

Concentrate is the cheapest of them all but can sometimes cause bloating if you buy the *really* cheap stuff. Hydrolsate absorbs the quickest. Which one should you buy? Whichever floats your boat. I usually go for isolate but at times I also buy "blends" which contain all three. Instead of getting all anal, I suggest you find a brand/product which you love, and will stick to.

## Protein (Casein)

This is a type of protein found in mammal milk; Casein makes up about 20-30% of human milk, and about 80% of cow's milk. It's also a vital component in making glue and serves as the industry standard when it comes to "slow releasing" proteins. Which means it's usually taken before bedtime so that it can be absorbed as you sleep – which is completely unnecessary in my opinion. You can take whey before bedtime and still experience a boost in recovery[5-11].

So why would you want a slow ass protein that is sticky and gel-like enough to be used in some of the strongest bonding glues in the world? Because, muscles. Actually casein is not only a great source of calcium and glutamine, but it doesn't become gel-like in your stomach when you take it. The marketed "slow absorption" happens in the intestines, not your stomach; casein passes through your stomach at a fairly decent pace.

You want casein in conjunction with whey made with good ol' milk. All 3 types of proteins are good on their own, but the whole is greater than the sum of the parts. A 20/50/30 percent blend, respectively, is something you can make over at truenutrition.com and I've been more than happy with the results. Also, use the premium flavouring – you'll thank me later.

"What about buying Milk, Egg and Beef protein powders?" If you're buying protein powder, it better be whey, casein or some permutation of the two. Only retards spend money on the other kinds. If you want protein from milk, eggs and beef... then drink milk, have some eggs and chew on a steak, damn it!

"What about soy?" I'll let one of my influencers tackle this one, "Soy is for dorks" – C.Poliquin. There, couldn't have said it better myself.

"But, I'm vegan!"

Then become un-vegan. You're not doing the world, or yourself any favours by going vegan. Vegetables and plants are basically carnivorous; friendly microorganisms that "work" for the plant, *kill* other organisms in the dirt and liquefy them into a nice bug juice which the plants then get to suck up through their roots. This is how they get their nutrients from soil. Then you come along with your hippie ways, and eat these plants.

So basically, instead of eating big animals, you're just eating little animals that have been pre-killed and pre-digested for you[5-12]. What, you mad? Good. Another reason to consider carnivore-ism is that meat eaters on the general have higher levels of growth hormone (GH) in their bodies than vegans – and GH does a whole bunch of awesome things such as: increase muscle mass, strength and oh yes, help with fat loss!

At the very least, consider becoming vegetarian so you can have milk and eggs because buying this book for the purposes of becoming shredded, then having a strong stance on being vegan is like handing me a fucking screw driver and asking me to build you a house. Sure, it can be done, but it'll take way too much effort and an ass load of time. Why wouldn't you instead use every tool available at your disposal?

**Recommended dosage:** There is none; whey protein is a convenience tool, so take your protein requirement which you calculated in chapter 3 and substitute as many grams as needed, depending on the busyness of your lifestyle. Generally speaking, whey shouldn't make up for more than 50% of your total daily protein intake. Not when the world has steak and bacon to offer.

## Creatine

This is one of the most heavily researched supplements on the market today, and for good reason – it works. Exercise recovery, assisting in lean muscle gains, improving strength and even aiding fat loss, creatine does it all (it's probably bff with fish oils). It's important to know that creatine is naturally occurring in meats, so even if you don't take the supplement, you'll still be getting some of it if you eat ample amounts of animal.

There are a few different types of creatine available but 99% of the time, you shouldn't bother with them; because the original form (creatine monohydrate) is still the undisputed king. It has out-performed some of the most popular types[5-21] and is generally cheaper to buy. In fact, most other creatine formulas are some form of lame imitation or permutation of monohydrate anyways. Some of the famous drawbacks of creatine are stomach bloating and/or water retention.

However, I've noticed that this is a rare occurrence and is usually more pronounced when you buy the cheap stuff. The highest quality monohydrate you can buy is CreaPure; it's made in Germany and has no imitators.  Buy it, and you should be fine ( **link:** http://www.fitjerk.com/creapure )
"What about the 1%?", you ask. Well there is another form of creatine called magnesium chelate (CMC). It's is basically creatine that has been attached to a bit of magnesium.

So while traditional creatine mohohydrate enters your cells using a sodium-dependant transporter, CMC finds a secondary pathway. A side-door entrance, if you will. In theory, it sounds nice and it might, on some random level, work better for you.
But in reality, there exists no conclusive scientific evidence that proves creatine magnesium chelate is superior to creatine monohydrate.

There is a study out there, which is being mentioned by the few companies marketing magnesium chelate to prove its superiority. But those studies compared CMC to magnesium oxide creatine (which sucks). So obviously, CMC outperformed it and now they brag like they've found the next best thing. But that's hardly a fair comparison; it would be like setting up a fight between The Hulk and Loki.

You don't need to conduct "experiments" or do any form of "science" to predict an accurate outcome. (If you didn't get that reference, you really need to go watch *The Avengers*, like, immediately.)

**Recommended dosage:** This is another area where there is lots of debate. Some say you should cycle it because constant use will damage your liver and kidneys. Others say it doesn't matter and you should take as much as you can. The truth, as always, lies somewhere in the middle of the two extremes. I've been taking creatine almost daily (in all different forms due to companies sending me stuff to review) for the better part of 5 years. No kidney, liver or excretion problems to report.

Now, is it a good idea to take a week or two off after a couple months? Yeah, it never hurts. Creatine *does* need to be loaded so if it's your first time, take 10-15g/day for the first week, then taper off to 5g/day thereafter.

This is the optimal scenario, and you can just as well start taking 5g/day everyday for a long time and still reap the benefits. As for timing, I recommend 2.5g pre and post workout. If you're a bigger individual (closer to 200lbs), then 5g pre and post workout should suffice. These doses are on the lower end and you can take more (that's your choice), but just remember that there's a cut off point where more creatine will not be absorbed by the body, and you'll literally be pissing away money.

## Beta-Alanine (BetaA)

Here's a simplistic explanation of how it works: People who generally lift heavy ass things at high intensities tend to have higher levels of carnosine in their muscles. Carnosine is basically a joint molecule which contains beta-alanine and histidine. It is found in high concentrations in muscle tissue and the brain. Those that have above-average carnosine levels in their muscles are able to prevent the drop in pH (since carnosine buffers H+ ions), this delays lactic acid build up (the burn you feel), which allows them to crank out more reps. More reps = more work done = better and faster results, generally speaking. But, there is a point where your natural carnosine levels will plateau, even if you've been training for years and the only way to increase them is by supplementation.

This is where BetaA comes in. BetaA is a precursor to carnosine synthesis, and it's also "rate limiting"... which means your levels of carnosine are limited by the amount of available BetaA. So when you take some BetaA orally, you increase your levels of muscle carnosine, allowing you to do more work[5-13] at a higher intensity[5-15].

BetaA is also the perfect example of the Supplement Reward Principal in effect – the stronger and leaner you are, the better it seems to work. So in theory, stacking this bad boy with creatine seems like a match made in heaven. And it sort of is.

**Recommended dosage:** Like creatine, BetaA needs to be loaded first in order to be effective, but the more BetaA you take, the more you start to piss out[5-14]. So start with 10g/day for one week, then use 5g/day on training days *only*, taken as a pre-workout. Just a word of warning: Be prepared for the BetaA "flush", or also known as "why do I feel like scratching my head and ass at the same time?"

Depending on the individual, the effects of the flush can range from mild skin tingles to the pins and needles feeling you get when you sleep on your arm for too long.

Don't freak out – that's pretty much what's supposed to happen. The precise reason as to why BetaA gives you the tingles isn't known, but one theory suggests that BetaA binds to nerve receptors which are situated right below the skin.

When it does this, it excites them to the point where they start firing off at random intervals; hence the tingles. When getting BetaA, I'd seriously invest in a back-scratcher simultaneously. In fact, I think I might start writing to supplement companies and demand they start selling it as a bundle deal.

And if all of this itching and scratching business bothers you (it's really not that bad), you may ditch the loading phase and just start taking 5g/day on training days only. Since this method isn't optimal, it will take a week or two for the effects of BetaA to work in your favour, so stack it with creatine. Oh, and you'll still feel the flush, but it should be less intense.

*Side Note: If you're looking for a decent product on the market, Cell Rush by AAEFX happens to be the best (and most economical) BetaA+Creatine product I've used thus far. 1-2 tablespoons and most people will feel it. You can read my full review here. While I am currently sponsored under AAEFX, back when I reveiwed CellRush I wasn't – it just happens to be a good product that I highly recommend. If you happen to have the printed copy of the book, visit http://www.fitjerk.com/cellrush*

## Caffeine

Ya can't have a fat loss book without talking about the most used (and probably abused) stimulant in all of human history, caffeine. It continues to surprise me with its sheer vast of abilities - it isn't just used as a 'pick me up' anymore. Nowadays, caffeine can help aid in fat loss due to its thermogenic properties[5-20], reduce muscle pain[5-16], decrease recovery times, suppress appetite, improve performance when you're feeling weak[5-19], and even increase work capacity[5-17].

Stack it with creatine+BetaA, and you'll have quite the powerful pre-workout performance enhancer on your hands[5-18]. It's not a bad recovery agent either. In fact, the CBC stack (Caffeine, BetaA, Creatine) is one of my personal favourites since it can literally pick me up by my undies, and get my caramel colored behind into the gym on days where I feel like vegetating on a couch.

The problem with caffeine though, is if you take too much constantly, you become resistant to it. This means you'll need a bigger dose to feel its effects. It's like dating a model; feels exciting for the first few months since she is hot as hell, but half a year in, you're already accustomed to her beauty and she needs to do a lot more than throw a smile on her pretty face to keep your attention.

Oh, never dated a model before? Just take my word for it, caffeine and models work in very similar ways. This trend of taking more caffeine can continue upwards at dangerous levels if you're not careful. Thankfully, taking about 2-4 weeks off can bring your caffeine sensitivity levels back to (somewhat) normal levels. If you're a hard-core stimulant junkie, you might need a bigger break than that.

**Recommended Dosage:** Take about 200-400mg per day. Ideally, I take about 100mg in the morning, which is my dark roast coffee, then about 200-300mg pre workout along with my creatine.

The CBC stack should be used as needed; don't take it for the sake of taking it. If you're highly caffeine sensitive (check with your doctor), then start with very tiny doses (50-100mg) and work your way up.

If you ever do a seriously grueling workout and feel that your ass got handed to you on a silver platter, then 200mg post workout can be a very good idea for recovery purposes. The golden rule is to not exceed 400-500mg in any given day.

**Fish Oils**

There is nothing fish oils can't do. Seriously, I've stopped reading research on it because the list of benefits are so vast, it comes across as the typical too-good-to-be-true scam.

Reduce inflammation? Done[5-3].

Reduce risk of heart disease? Done[5-4].

Improve joint function and mobility? Done[5-5].

Facilitate fat loss? Sure[5-6].

Increase strength? You betcha[5-7]!

Make you more anabolic? Duh[5-8].

Improve immune function? Most probably[5-9].

In fact, I've come up with my very own fish oil game. It's called "I want this benefit." Let's play. Go ahead, give me a benefit that you want, any benefit. The more ridiculous, the better. Got one? Good. Want to know how to achieve this benefit?

Take fish oils[5-10].

Go ahead, think of another. Oh, you want psychic powers?

Take fish oils[5-10].

See, don't ever say FJ didn't make learning fun.

**Recommended dose:** Take 1-2 tbsp daily, forever. In fact even after you die, tell them to pour fish oil over your body, since it's probably also a very good preservative. This way, your loved ones can admire your flawless physical appearance.

Some of you might think that taking straight oil is weird, and it is if you buy complete crap.

Personally, I recommend the stuff from Ascenta (visit: www.fitjerk.com/fishoil) which has a hint of lemon flavour and goes down with minimal fuss, especially when chased with some orange juice.

---

5-10: All joking aside, while the benefits of fish oils are numerous, it's not the end all be all. Taking it won't solve all your problems and there is just as much neutral evidence as there is positive. Like most substances, its effectiveness ends up standing on middle ground, and so should you. Taking the listed dose, combined with the effective exercise program will provide positive health benefits, but don't try and over-compensate by taking more of it. More is not always better – even water can be toxic at the right dose.

## Vitamin D

Sunscreen, video games, the lure of indoor convenience and the rise of dumbshit vampire soap operas are just a few of the reasons why the North American population is ridiculously deficient in Vitamin D. And this causes everyone to become miserable, fat and lethargic. Fellas, the next time a lady is rude to you at the bar, don't call her a "bitch", the poor girl is probably just Vitamin D deficient.

Tell her, you'll show her something called "the sun", it's a sure thing. Ladies, you'll know your man is deficient if he can't, ahem, perform aptly. Before swinging for the tiny blue pills, reach for Vitamin D tabs (plus some Yohimbine HCL) and use em to spike everything he ingests.

What's more, every part of your body needs Vitmain D for optimal functioning; without it, your metabolic rate will suffer, your energy levels will be all out of whack, insulin sensitivity will go out the window, you'll start to feel hungry for no apparent reason, and fat will infiltrate your muscles[5-22] like a SWAT team with bad intentions.

Another problem seems to be that the general recommended daily dosage of Vitmain D is too low. So we have "experts" and "health organizations" that are telling people that they need X amount, when in reality they need about 5X or even 10X[5-23].

So we have people who are already walking around with low Vitamin D levels, not taking enough because they are being told that what they need is about 5-10 times less. This is like accidentally setting a kitten on fire, then trying to put it out with a fork. And I like kittens, so that was more painful for me to type, than for you to visualize.

Having said all of that, know that taking Vitamin D doesn't affect fat loss directly - it's not a thermogenic like caffeine. If you take enough, what it will do is make sure that your body is functioning optimally so that you either return to your regular body fat levels, or have a much easier time losing fat when a proper plan is in place. It's like removing the monkey wrench stuck inside a giant malfunctioning machine, then greasing it – so it'll work as intended, but not much better.

**Recommended Dosage:** Depending on your activity levels, where you live (sunny or not so sunny) and how often you go outside, taking anywhere from 2000-4000 IU per day should be sufficient. You can even cycle it and take more on training days and less on rest days. Also, worrying about overdose is not an issue since like most people, you're probably deficient anyways, but try and stay under 5000-7000 IU.

## Yohimbine HCL (YHCL)

Basically a stimulant which is prescribed (in pure form) to treat impotence in men. Also seems to elicit anti-depressant qualities, and has been used to boost blood pressure, so you want lean on the side of caution. However, our concern is fat loss not sexual setbacks, and in that sense YHCL seems promising.

There was a study[5-24] done on 20 soccer players where one group took 20 milligrams of YHCL per day for 21 days and the placebo group took cellulose. While there were no differences in body mass or muscle mass, the YHCL group lost a bit of fat by the end of the trail and it seems as if though they maintained this during the post-supplementation assessment.

Performance on the other hand stayed the same, and no side effects were reported by the soccer players. While this makes YHCL sound like the holy grail of fat loss solutions, you need to be aware of one important factor: the test subjects were elite soccer players, which means it's not a stretch to assume they were on gruelling workout programs and already in good shape.

This means their bodies probably had better blood flow than the average person. And since YHCL seems to work by increasing blood flow to the fat cells, the dramatic results all make sense. The soccer player study may be another example of the Supplement Reward Principal in effect.

**Recommended dosage:** The dose that the soccer players took at 21mg is considered a bit high. I would start at 5mg/day and slowly work my way up since it YHCL does become more effective as it gets loaded. If 5mg/day for a week or so shows no side effects, you can bump it to 10mg/day. Personally, I wouldn't go higher than that. As far as timing is concerned, I haven't read anything that shows there's an optimal time to take it, but since it's a stimulant, use it in the morning or whenever you need slight kick in the ass to get going.

Oh, and I assume you've read the disclaimer presented at the start of this book, but it bears repeating that you should be careful with YHCL. Do-not-fuck around and assume you can take the dose mentioned in the study. I shall **not** be responsible for your brainless dumbassery should you hurt yourself.

# Chapter 5 References

5-1: *Grew Up A Screw Up – Ludacris*

5-2: **Placebos Are Getting More Effective. Drugmakers Are Desperate to Know Why.**

5-3: **Omega-3 fatty acids EPA and DHA: health benefits throughout life**

5-4: **Omega-3 fatty acids in high-risk cardiovascular patients: a meta-analysis of randomized controlled trials**

5-5: **A randomized, double-blinded, placebo-controlled study of the effect of a combination of lemon verbena extract and fish oil omega-3 fatty acid on joint management**

5-6: **Combining fish-oil supplements with regular aerobic exercise improves body composition and cardiovascular disease risk factors.**

5-7: **Fish-oil supplementation enhances the effects of strength training in elderly women**

5-8: **Omega-3 polyunsaturated fatty acids augment the muscle protein anabolic response to hyperinsulinaemia-hyperaminoacidaemia in healthy young and middle-aged men and women**

5-9: **Effect of fish oil diet on immune response and proteinuria in mice**

5-11: **Protein Ingestion Prior To Sleep Improves Post-Exercise Overnight Recovery**

5-12: **Nutrition: The Dirt Facts** by Paul Chek

5-13: **beta-Alanine supplementation augments muscle carnosine content and attenuates fatigue during repeated isokinetic contraction bouts in trained sprinters.**

5-14: **The absorption of orally supplied beta-alanine and its effect on muscle carnosine synthesis in human vastus lateralis.**

5-15: **Ergogenic effects of betaine supplementation on strength and power performance.**

5-16: **Caffeine Reduces Muscle Pain From Exercise**

5-17: **Caffeine lowers muscle pain during exercise in hot but not cool environments**

5-18: **Ingesting a pre-workout supplement containing caffeine, B-vitamins, amino acids, creatine, and beta-alanine before exercise delays fatigue while improving reaction time and muscular endurance**

5-19: **Caffeine ingestion reverses the circadian rhythm effects on neuromuscular performance in highly resistance-trained men.**

5-20: **Comparison of changes in energy expenditure and body temperatures after caffeine consumption.**

5-21: **The effects of creatine ethyl ester supplementation combined with heavy resistance training on body composition, muscle performance, and serum and muscle creatine levels**

5-22: **Vitamin D status and its relation to muscle mass and muscle fat in young women.**

5-23: **Vitamin d: extraskeletal health.**

5-24: **Yohimbine: the effects on body composition and exercise performance in soccer players**

5-25: If you have the printed version of the book, my supplement reviews can be found here:

http://flawlessfitnessbook.com/blog/category/reviews/supplement-reviews/

# Chapter 6: Its Showtime
# (Putting It All Together)

# Stage 1 Fat Loss Plan (General Deficit)

If you're at a body fat level of 15% or higher, then this is where you start. If you're not, move to stage 2. There are two main reasons for the stage 1 plan:

1. **To help build discipline and get you used to being on a meal plan**
2. **To help you through the "easy" stage of fat loss (visceral)**

Do not underestimate the importance of those two reasons; jumping into stage 2 without such prerequisites will feel like being tossed inside a shark tank. If you're not up for it, you'll be eaten alive. The stage 1 process will also help you work out any quirks and you'll get to know your preferences rather well. For example, do you prefer to make your chicken in advance and freeze it? Or do you prefer to make it as needed and keep a huge stash in your fridge?

You need to find what works with your lifestyle and the only way to do this, is by trial and error. The stage 1 plan is also a good place to make mistakes and learn from them, as the margin for error in the stage 2 plan is razor thin. So here we go...

### Step 1: Find And Test Your BMR

I covered this in great detail in chapter 3. If you haven't done your calculations by now, go ahead and do so. Test it out till you know your exact BMR value.

### Step 2: Finding Your Training & Resting Day Calories

Once you have your BMR, you need to subtract it by two numbers, 250 and 500. The (BMR-250) number is the amount of calories you'll take in during your training day, and (BMR-500) is the number of calories you'll be taking in on rest days. The number of workout days and rest days will depend on the workout plan you create and/or choose.

If you find that your weight doesn't change or rate of fat loss isn't satisfactory, use (BMR-500) for both days while still using the macro ratios listed below. If that doesn't work, it means your BMR was incorrect, so subtract further.

## Step 3: Picking Your Macro Ratios

For the rest days, use macro ratio percentages of 45/25/30 (protein, carbs & fats respectively) and for the training days, use macro ratio percentages of 35/50/15 (protein, carbs & fats respectively). You should already know how to divide these up but for the sake of clarity, below is an example of the first ratio. Remember that protein and carbs = 4 calories per gram and fat = 9 calories per gram.

**BMR** = 2100 calories
**Protein:** (2100 x 0.45)/4 = 236.25 grams
**Carbs:** (2100 x 0.25)/4 = 131.25 grams
**Fats:** (2100 x 0.30)/9 = 70 grams

## Step 4: Devise Or Pick A Workout Plan

Use the exercise list in chapter 4 and the workout template in chapter 7 to create your very own workout plan. Or, you can use the custom workout routines already created for you in chapter 7. Either way, be sure to bust some serious ass when you do these workouts. As far as frequency is concerned, 3x a week is the bare minimum.

## (Optional): Pick Your Supplements

You now know what supplements I recommend and their dosages. Combine them with your meal plan if you wish. I highly suggest basics ones such as multivitamin, caffeine and protein. Everything else is your choice. Don't ask me if you should take YHCL. You have the facts, so make your own damn decisions.

Now, below are 3 examples of what your diet outline will look like. The first plan meets the bare minimum requirements; the next one is a more hardcore version and the final one incorporates a fasting protocol. Another thing I want you to remember is to stay *consistent* with your workouts while practicing progressive overload.

So if you follow the first example below, do the exact same GDW (glycogen depletion workout) that you did on Monday and Wednesday for 4-6 weeks but lift heavier weights as the weeks go on. Don't lift the same crap over and over again for too long – your body will get used to it, your progress *will* stall, and you *will* cry.

**GDW** = Glycogen Depletion Workout
**ST** = Strength Training Workout
**IC** = Interval Cardio

## Stage 1 Bare Minimum | Weekly Caloric Deficit From Diet: 2750

| Monday | Tuesday | Wednesday | Thursday | Friday | Saturday | Sunday |
|--------|---------|-----------|----------|--------|----------|--------|
| BMR-250 | BMR-500 | BMR-250 | BMR-500 | BMR-250 | BMR-500 | BMR-500 |
| GDW | Rest | GDW | Rest | ST | Rest | Rest |

## Stage 1 Quite Maximum | Weekly Caloric Deficit From Diet: 2500

| Monday | Tuesday | Wednesday | Thursday | Friday | Saturday | Sunday |
|--------|---------|-----------|----------|--------|----------|--------|
| BMR-250 | BMR-500 | BMR-250 | BMR-500 | BMR-250 | BMR-250 | BMR-500 |
| GDW | IC | ST | IC | GDW | ST | IC |

You might be wondering why the person in the 2nd example would be following the BMR-500 meal plan on the cardio days. And the reason is simple: cardio workouts are just not as demanding as the others, so taking a bigger caloric hit is fine. You'll more than survive.

## For The Ifast Crowd

If you want to practice fasting, you may replace any one of the BMR-500 days with a full 24 hour fast and workout days with your maintenance (BMR) calories. However, don't bother doing more than 2 fasts per week. Below is an example week of someone who wants to follow a fasting protocol while doing the Stage 1 Fat Loss Plan

## Stage 1 With Ifast | Weekly Caloric Deficit From Diet: (BMR x 2) + 1000

| Monday | Tuesday | Wednesday | Thursday | Friday | Saturday | Sunday |
|--------|---------|-----------|----------|--------|----------|--------|
| BMR | Fast | BMR | Fast | BMR | BMR-500 | BMR-500 |
| GDW | Rest | GDW | Rest | ST | Rest | Rest |

# Stage 2 Fat Loss Plan (Carb Cycling)

This is when things start to get fun, and by fun, I mean testing the limits of your will power and sanity. Truth be told, if you keep yourself busy and call on the aid of the appropriate supplements, then it's really not that bad.

You'll basically have four meal plans: lowcarb40(LC40), lowcarb50(LC50), high carb(HC) and maintenance (which is basically your BMR). When possible, be sure to use the meal and feeding timings to your advantage:

- Most (60-80%) of carbs should be eaten post workout
- You must take in some protein pre & post workout
- Try and consume most of your calories by night time

**Step 1: Chart Out Your Week**
If you're doing the stage 2 fat loss plan, then I assume you're somewhere around 15% bodyfat. Below are two examples of what a carb-cycling week should look like, but depending on your lifestyle you might have to change things around.

This is fine, but the maintenance and high carb days must be together as listed and you need two LC40 and two LC50 days in the plan. Calculating the "LC" plans will be explained below...

| Monday | Tuesday | Wednesday | Thursday | Friday | Saturday | Sunday |
|--------|---------|-----------|----------|--------|----------|--------|
| LC40 | LC40 | LC50 | LC50 | Maintenance | HC | Maintenance |

Another example could be...

| Monday | Tuesday | Wednesday | Thursday | Friday | Saturday | Sunday |
|--------|---------|-----------|----------|--------|----------|--------|
| Maintenance | HC | Maintenance | LC50 | LC50 | LC40 | LC40 |

## Step 2: Figure Out Your Low Carb Numbers

Take your BMR, divide it in half and write it down that number. Then take your BMR, multiply it by 0.4 and write that down as well. The first number is the amount of calories you'll consume during the LC50 days, and the latter during the LC40 days. So if your BMR is 2000, the total food you'll consume on your LC50 days will be 1000 calories, and 800 calories during LC40 days.

Now that you have your calories, you need to divide them up so you know how much protein, carbs and fats to stuff your face with. Doing this is easy; pick your favorite macro ratio from Chpater 3 and split it all up. You can use the same macro ratio for both LC40 and LC50 or mix things up. Your choice.

Personally to keep things simple, I'd pick one macro ratio and stick with it.

## Step 3: Find Out Your High Carb Numbers

Take your BMR and multiply this by 1.75, which will give you the amount of calories to eat on your high carb days. So for example, if your BMR was 2000 calories, then on your high carb days, you would be taking in 3500 calories. When it comes to your macros, the only important one is protein – keep this at 20% minimum, and the rest is up to you.

Want to eat fatty foods? Awesome, go for it.

Are you more of a carb person? Perfect, that works too.

High carb days are your time to indulge, so make sure you do so. If you've worked hard during the week, then you've earned the right.

## Step 4: Figure Out Your Training

The amount that you train is up to you, but there are certain rules to follow that I've listed below.

- **Minimum of 3 workouts per week**
- Do glycogen depletion on low carb days (light load, reps: 15-20 range and sets: 3-4 range)
- Do strength training during high carb or maintenance days (heavy load, reps: 3-5 range, sets: 5-10 range)
- If you feel like training 2x a day, leave a 6-8 hour gap between the two workouts
- Cardio workouts can be done whenever, as long as they don't break rule #4
- There is no maximum; you can do multiple workouts a day if you're feeling hardcore, as long as you don't break rule #4
- Your workouts should be intense and under 60 minutes long
- Do not go to failure; leave a rep or two in the gas tank regardless of the workout

Below are two examples of what a week might look like. The top row is the meal plan, and the bottom row is the workout plan. The plan in the first week meets the bare minimum requirements and the latter is for someone who wants to see results quickly... such as dropping up to 5lbs in a week type quickly.

**Legend**
GDW = Glycogen Depletion Workout | ST = Strength Training Workout | IC = Interval Cardio

## The Sane

| Monday | Tuesday | Wednesday | Thursday | Friday | Saturday | Sunday |
|--------|---------|-----------|----------|--------|----------|--------|
| LC40 | LC40 | LC50 | LC50 | Maintenance | HC | Maintenance |
| GDW | Rest | IC | Rest | Rest | ST | Rest |

## The InSane

| Monday | Tuesday | Wednesday | Thursday | Friday | Saturday | Sunday |
|--------|---------|-----------|----------|--------|----------|--------|
| LC40 | LC40 | LC50 | LC50 | Maintenance | HC | Maintenance |
| IC am | IC | IC am | IC | IC am | ST am | IC am |
| GDW pm | | GDW pm | | ST pm | GDW pm | ST pm |

**Quick Notes & Tips:** Use supplements as necessary such as caffeine on Low Carb days to keep you from feeling tired. Coffee is a great idea and as far as I'm concerned, 2-3 cups a day is just fine.

Now, for the coffee haters out there who preposterously hate on this heavenly brew while claiming it's bad for you, let me enlighten your dumbasses: Coffee drinkers have it good in a multitude of ways[6-1,6-2], such as: less likely to have type 2 diabetes, Parkinson's disease, dementia, have fewer chances of heart problems, and lower risk of certain types of cancer such as prostate!

If a supplement company could come up with a product and rightfully claim such benefits, it would bring in billions. Also, use liquid substitutes such as protein shakes to meet the mountainous caloric requirements for the high carb days. Unless you're Furious Pete (pro speed eater), you'll most definitely need liquid assistance.

And finally, if you really want to accelerate results, you can replace one of your Maintenance days with an LC50 meal plan - as you can see, this shit is very scalable to the individual.

# Stage 3 – Fat Loss Maintenance With Fasting

If you recall from chapter 3, I said ifast is useful when needed, and I currently know of no better method which you can use to maintain your lean body, than ifast. Unless maybe copious amounts of sex while on a caloric deficit, but that is not a method easily accessible by all. So as you saw, we can incorporate ifast in stage 1 but if the mild side effects of fasting get to you, such as unbearable hunger pangs, headaches and or nausea, then you should probably stick to the general deficit and train your body to live off less calories first.

Once you have the discipline in place, I will say that after about a week or so on ifast, your body gets used to it and the inconveniences tend to be mild. It's only when you jump cold turkey into ifast that things get unpleasant – at least from the feedback I've gathered. And on a side note, incorporating ifast into stage 2 is completely out of the question, so don't even ask. That is a very specific protocol so do not mish-mash it with anything else. Now, back to fasting as a maintenance tool, let's begin...

**Step 1: Re-Calculate your BMR**
After achieving the body you want using Stage 1 and Stage 2 methods, chances are your BMR isn't the same anymore. In fact, it may have gone up even though your body weight has dropped. That's the beauty of having a high metabolism. So use the exact same methods you used previously, and calculate your new BMR. I'll call this new BMR value, "Z".

**Step 2: Select an ifast method**
You have two choices: either pick the simple method where you have three 24 hour fasts during the week or the advanced method which requires a daily 16 hour fast with an 8 hour feeding window. If you're choosing the simple method, then you'll need to make up for the deficit by spreading it out through the days where you aren't fasting.

For example, if your Z value is 2500 and you choose to do 3 fasts a week, then that is three days worth of calories (2500 x 3 = 7500) you'll have to spread out during the feeding days. Otherwise, you'll end up losing weight even further. If this is what you want then feel free. Below is what an example week with the calculated calories might look like...

| Monday | Tuesday | Wednesday | Thursday | Friday | Saturday | Sunday |
|---|---|---|---|---|---|---|
| Fast | Feed | Fast | Feed | Fast | Feed | Feed |
| 0 kcal | 5000 kcal | 0 kcal | 5000 kcal | 0 kcal | 5000 kcal | 2500 kcal |

Yeah I know what you're thinking, "How the hell am I supposed to take in 5000 calories on feeding day?!" Well, you freakin try. You've always wanted permission to pig out, right? So quit the bitchin' and start eating. And if you can't, then you can't. Remember that you're on maintenance, so as long as your total weekly intake is less or equal to the total weekly required (Z x 7), your weight shouldn't change.

It's also worth noting that three 24 hour fasts per week for maintenance might be an overkill and you should be fine with two. Still, you won't know till you play around with this so be willing to experiment. As for your macro breakdowns, pick one of the ones I mentioned in Chapter 3, or if you're feeling creative then come up with your own. As long as protein stays at 1.2g per pound of bodyweight you're currently at, you really can't go wrong.
When it comes to the advanced ifast method, the exact process was already discussed in the chapter 3 section *"On Fasting"*. All you have to do is use your newly adjusted BMR (Z value) for the calculations.

### What About Training On ifast Maintenance?

K.I.S.S* - Stick to GDW & Strength type workouts, 3-4 times per week. When you're on maintenance, you can stop worrying about crazy details and have some fun. Love doing curls? Go nuts. Want to do some CultFit... er, I mean CrossFit? Sure, break a leg. Literally[4-2].

Just make sure your progress isn't stagnating and you're lifting heavier and getting stronger as the weeks go by. So if you're doing your curls, make sure you aren't doing 50lbs for 3 sets of 7 for six weeks in a row. That is not maintaining, it's more like wasting your time. Calories can be maintained and kept the same for weeks, months or even years, but this rule *does not* apply to your workouts.

*K.I.S.S [kiss] – is an abbreviation for Keep It Simple, Stupid.*

# Take A Break

After about 8 weeks on any of the plans (excluding stage 3), take a week off and eat at maintenance (BMR) while keeping your workouts short, swift and sweet (20 minutes or less, regardless of IC, GDW or ST). Especially if you're doing stage 2, as going on such an extreme plan for a long time is mentally draining and will only be detrimental to your results if you push yourself too hard.

In fact, there was an interesting study[6-3] done where subjects on a diet were told to take a break for 2 weeks, and the assumption was, in that period of time they'll most likely balloon in size. Basically, the researchers were trying to see if throwing a monkey wrench (the 2 week break) into a structured weight loss plan would cause these people to relapse and suffer through a phenomenon known as "yo-yo" dieting. Or as I like to call it, "Kirstie Alley Syndrome".

But guess what happened? Their evil plan backfired and none of that yo-yo crap happened. In fact, the subjects not only *maintained* their general weight before going on the break, but they also had no troubles jumping right back into the diet and continuing where they left off. It was as if someone hit the "pause" button. Now think about the implications of what I just described... go ahead, let it sink in. What this means is, after every 6-8 weeks you essentially earn a "pause" button (or a "wild card"), which can be cashed in right before a vacation, family gathering, emergency etc. Convenient? You bet your right ass-cheek it is!

### Why Breaks Work

It all comes back to the same reasons I talked about in the *"Advanced Carb Cycling"* section in chapter 3. When you diet, regardless of how aggressive it is, your body is like, "wtf you doing?!" and tries to compensate accordingly.

This results in unwanted situations such as a drop in metabolic rate, hormone imbalance, low energy levels etc. So when you take a week off and just eat at maintenance, you give your body time to set the record straight by bringing your hormone levels back up to normal which makes you generally feel better – both mentally and physically.

Speaking of mentality, I think the psychological benefits behind a break are more important than the physiological, and it ties in with step 3 (small chunking goals) in my *"How To Set And Achieve Goals"* section in chapter 1. When you know you only have to follow your diet plan for 6-8 weeks instead of 15 or 20 weeks, it really takes the stress off things. Even if shit gets hard, you can remind yourself that there are only a few more weeks left, and that quitting is for pathetic little bitches, which you are most certainly *not*.

If and when you try the stage 2 plan, notice how good you end up getting at this "looking forward to a break" thing, since you already get one at the end of every week with the high carb day.

**How To Use Breaks Effectively**

While you might be gleaming with joy like a pre-school girl who's discovered a new found love for Barbie dolls about having your very own "pause" button, I need to throw down a mighty word of caution... actually, it's more like a sentence of caution but, whatever.

And it is this: **going on a break does not give you carte blanche to return to your old, crappy eating habits while living a life of immobility.** There is a reason I say eat maintenance on your break week and not, "whatever the fuck you want". If that doesn't make my point crystal clear, lord help you.

So, when and how do you know you're ready for a break? Easy, if you're on the stage 1 plan, take one every 8 weeks and if you're on the stage 2 plan, take one when you feel like it, but only after being on the plan for 6 weeks, minimum. So it can be after 6, 7, 8, 9 or even 10 weeks. And since there *are* some seriously tough willed individuals out there, I will say that you shouldn't go for more than 12 weeks on the stage 2 plan without going on a break. Mentally you might not need it because your level of willpower defies logic, but physiologically, you do.

What about breaks during the stage 3 plan? Well first, you need to understand it is specifically designed to be used for the long term. We're talking years to quite possibly the rest of your life. Yes, it truly is that sustainable. Having said that, you can still take a break during stage 3 to get away from fasting for a week or two, should you need it.

That's the beauty of success when it comes to fitness – once you've reached your desire state, maintenance is easier than picking up a cheap hooker with $100 bills taped to your forehead. The hard part is getting there.

# Strategies For Handling Holiday Temptations

Let's face it, no matter how many tricks, techniques and gadgets you learn about, putting in the hard ass work to burn calories is something you won't be able to get away from. That intense sensation of lactic acid is here to stay – and no magical wizardry is going to take it away or make it any easier. Which means you'll have to endure a bit of pain to get the result you want.

But here's the awesome thing about this type of pain (the pain of discipline) – it only lasts briefly; a few minutes, a few hours or even a few days. But the pain of discipline will always go away and will be replaced with a result. A result you earned and hopefully wanted.

However, on the flipside we have another type of pain – the one of regret. Initially this pain isn't as intense as the one mentioned above, but it's like a thorn stuck in your back that you can't reach. It will linger for a long, long time. The pain of regret is the feeling you get when a month later you say to yourself, "damn, if only I started going to the gym consistently... I would be like 10lbs lighter by now!"

And at this point, when the digotal book has just been published (5 months into 2012), I can pretty much guarantee there's a boat load of people feeling an enormous amount of pain from regret. And the sad part is that it could have been prevented. If only they weren't such panzies and endured the short term pain and did what they were supposed to do. If only.

But you can't go back and change history. The only way to trump the pain of regret is to take action... and take it enough times so that your achievements will dwarf the moments when you chose to sit on the couch and do jack all. So as we slowly approach the holiday season of 2012, here are my top 3 tips that will prevent you from feeling the pain of regret.

## 1. Don't Wait For New Years

Making yearly health and fitness resolutions is an act of stupidity that cannot be fathomed by me. But I try. Never, ever wait for new years to make a resolution. Time itself doesn't give a shit whether it's new years or not; it will always keep moving forward. There is no next year, last year, tomorrow or yesterday. There is just today, and this moment. If your plan was to read this book, then maybe a few months down the road take some kind of action, then I say you stop, and take action *now*. As in, as soon as you finish reading the final sentence on the last page. Get at it, sucker!

## 2. How And When To Say "NO!" To Pressure From Others

Your family won't hate you. You'll still have friends. Your spouse won't leave you. Your dog won't die. And the world will not come to an end – you're not that important. All of these things are self-fulfilling prophecies that you bring into reality by believing they will come true if you say "no". Look, if you say "no" like a total loser, people will treat you like one and will keep pushing forward.

When I say "no" it's as definitive and authoritative as it gets – which means people know I mean it. I don't come across as an asshole, it's just that when I say no, it means fucking NO... and people around me respect that. If they don't, then I don't deal with them and are ignored from my life. Simple.

Now learning *how* to say "no" is only half the battle - the other half is knowing *when* to say "no". This means you should have a handle on which types of foods should enter your mouth and which ones shouldn't. And since I don't want to turn you into some nutritional robot during festive feats, my rule is simple – enjoy everything, but bust out the "no" when the portion starts to increase.

Want some cake that obviously looks like it will go to your ass? Sure, just cut the slice in half. Want to have wine? Sure, have "a" glass then say no. Get what I'm saying? Cut yourself off (and cut off others) when you're being fed more than you should be eating. Using your fist as a measure of portion size is very useful, as is using it to punch certain people when they frustrate and constantly harass you. I'm not saying you should... I'm just saying you *could*.

### 3. Reallocate Resources

Ok, so it's Christmas morning and after opening all your presents you realize that at the end of the day, there's gonna be a huge family dinner where you'll have a tough time saying "no" because you're weak. No problem, at least you're admitting it. But I've got a trick up my sleeve and it's a suggestion I give to my E-Training clients all the time. What you do is eat one meal after doing a small 30 minute workout in the morning (at home, since most gyms probably won't be open) and then stay away from food for the rest of the day, until dinner time.

Since you're taking in calories after a high intensity workout, it will be nearly impossible for your body to store it as fat, and your metabolic rate will be on fire for the rest of the day. For the average person, this little trick should result in an easy 1000 calorie deficit. Sometimes more.

It's like doing a mini fast. Or if you're already on one of the fasting protocols, you can time it so that the feast ends up being your fast breaker. The best part is that when dinner time rolls around, you can usually let lose (but not get out-of-control). Because of the huge deficit that you endured during the day, you'll find that after the dinner you're probably on track and haven't gone over your set limits (assuming you've already calculated them).

So there you go – three easy little tricks you can use to keep yourself in check during the insane holiday season. Do yourself a favor and make sure you take action as soon as you're done reading my brilliance. Don't be one of those people who looks back and says to themselves, "if only..."

Screw "if only..." and instead adopt the phrase, "I'm so glad I did..."

It's a much better feeling – trust me on this.

# Chapter 6 References

6-1: **Coffee And Your Health**

6-2: **Coffee consumption and prostate cancer risk and progression in the Health Professionals Follow-up Study**

6-3: **Prescribed "breaks" as a means to disrupt weight control efforts**

# Chapter 7: I Have Taught You How To Fish… But Fuck It, Here Is Some Salmon Too (Resources)

# Meal Plan Templates

Below are a few pre-made meal plan templates I've included and should cover quite the range of caloric requirements. Once you find your BMR and macros, adjust the plans below to suit your needs. These plans are meant to be used as templates, so you don't have to start from scratch. If you want to know how much protein, carbs and fat a certain type of food is made up of, you can visit a plethora of websites that will give you this information. One of them is http://nutritiondata.self.com/

For example, a skinless chicken breast has about 30g of protein, 0g of carbs and 2g of fat. If you were to remove this item from Meal Plan 2, you would end up with a total of 145g of protein, 42g of carbs and 58g of fat. Pretty straight forward stuff.

**Meal Plan 1**
2 Eggs
1 Packet Instant Quaker Oatmeal
3 Scoops Whey Protein
2 Cups Raw Vegetables And/Or Fruits

Total Protein: 96g
Total Carbs: 62g
Total Fat: 23g
Total Calories: 839

**Meal Plan 2**
2 Scoops Whey Protein ISOLATE
1 Skinless Chicken Breast
7oz Lean Ground Beef 90% (cooked how you like)
3 Cups Mixed Vegetables (RAW & Uncooked if possible)
1/2 Cup Frozen Yogurt (Fruit based flavor ONLY)
1/2 Tbsp Butter (Use it to cook or melt on veggies with spices)
7oz Beef Steak

Total Protein: 175g
Total Carbs: 42g
Total Fat: 60g
Total Calories: 1410

## Meal Plan 3
2 Scoops Gold Standard Whey Protein
1 Packet Quaker Instant Oatmeal
4oz Cooked Pasta
1/2 Cup Pasta Sauce
6oz Turkey (Ground or Breast)
1 Cup Cooked Brown Rice
1 Skinless Chicken Breast
1 Can chunk white tuna
4 Eggs
Total Protein: 207g
Total Carbs: 169g
Total Fat: 40.50g
Total Calories: 1868

## Meal Plan 4
2 Tbsp Jam
3 Slices Whole Wheat Toast
2 Skinless Chicken Breasts
1 Can Tuna (Cooked or Straight)
6 Cups Mixed Raw Veggies (Or slightly cook/steamed)
2 Packets Quaker Instant Oatmeal
6oz Turkey Breast (Or Ground)
4 Cups Mashed Potatoes w/butter
2 Cups Cooked Brown Rice
2 Cups Frosted Mini Wheats + Milk
2 Scoops Whey Protein Isolate
4oz Cooked Pasta + Sauce
Total Protein: 279g
Total Carbs: 550g
Total Fat: 55.50g
Total Calories: 3815.50

**Create Your Own Meal Plan:**

- 
- 
- 
- 
- 
- 
- 
- 

Total Protein:
Total Carbs:
Total Fat:
Total Calories:

**Create Your Own Meal Plan:**

- 
- 
- 
- 
- 
- 
- 
- 

Total Protein:
Total Carbs:
Total Fat:
Total Calories:

# Workout Templates

Like the meal plan templates, these are to be edited if and when needed. Before we get into the templates, I want to give you some general guidelines and rules of thumb on how to create your own using the exercise list in Chapter 4.

1. Exercises that involve the largest number of muscle groups come first (e.g squats before calf raises).
2. Barbell exercises are to be done before dumbbell exercises as long as rule #1 isn't broken.

Stack excises in either push/pull fashion (also known as protagonist/antagonist) such as bench press followed by pendlay rows or stick to one type of movement and follow rule number 1 & 2 such as having a pull only day, where you'd start with deadlifts and end with something like DB rows.

If there is a "tie" (such as between deadlifts and powercleans), then the more dynamic exercise, which is the powerclean in this case, would come first. If you're not dealing with dynamic exercises then the general order is this: Squats > Bench Press > Deadlifts

- Warm ups should be exercise specific, so if you're about to bench, do 8-10 reps with the bar and another set with really light loads (30-40% 1RM). You can even do a few sets of pushups. Literally anything that will get the blood flowing and will lubricate the joints is a good thing.

These general rules should serve you well but remember, rules exist so you know when to break them. The reason we squat before deadlifts is because the deadlift completely exhausts your lower back. So squatting right after such a situation (where the pre-exhausted lower back can post a bottle neck) is a good way to get injured - or feel like you've joined up for a CrossFit class.

But there are times when people will be using the squat rack (rare, but it happens) and you just won't have time to wait around. Not a problem, you have three choices:

1, Do your deadlifts and then take a huge break in between so your lower back has time to recover. 2, Squat another day. Or 3, sandwich your squat workout - so you'd deadlift for a few sets till the squat rack is free, do your squats, then get back to the deadlift. I've had to resort to all three of these options in the past, and they've served me well.

## Legend
BB = Barbells
DB = Dumbbells
BW = BodyWeight
GDW = Glycogen Depletion Workout
ST = Strength Training Workout
# = As many reps as possible, but not to failure

**Note:** Some workouts can have dual personalities and be used as GDW or ST. This optional change is listed in brackets. So if a listed GDW workout can be used for strength training, you'll see "(ST)". If you recall, all you have to do is adjust the load, rep range and rest time in between the exercises to make the changes.

### Workout 1 ST (GDW) | Rest: 60-180 seconds

| Exercise | Reps | Sets | Tempo | Lbs |
|---|---|---|---|---|
| BB Parallel Squat | 3 | 8 | 20X | |
| BB Full ROM Squat | 5 | 4 | 20X | |
| DB Step Ups | 8 | 3 | 10X | |
| Glute Ham Raise | 8 | 3 | 31X | |
| Calf Raises | 12-15 | 3 | 10X | |

### Workout 2 ST (GDW)| Rest: 60-180 seconds

| Exercise | Reps | Sets | Tempo | Lbs |
|---|---|---|---|---|

| BB Bench Press | 3 | 8 | 21X | |
|---|---|---|---|---|
| BB Overhead Press | 5 | 4 | 20X | |
| BB Close Grip Bench | 8 | 3 | 31X | |
| DB Incline Bench | 10 | 3 | 31X | |
| DB External Rotator Cuff | 10-12 | 3 | 311 | |

## Workout 3 ST (GDW) | Rest: 60-180 seconds

| Exercise | Reps | Sets | Tempo | Lbs |
|---|---|---|---|---|
| BB Deadlift | 3 | 8 | 21X | |
| Stiff Leg Rack Pulls | 5 | 4 | 21X | |
| Suitcase Deadlifts | 5 | 4 | 21X | |
| BB Hip Thrusts | 8 | 3 | 21X | |
| Hyper Extensions | 10-12 | 3 | 31X | |

## Workout 4 GDW beginner | Rest: 45 seconds

| Exercise | Reps | Sets | Tempo | Lbs |
|---|---|---|---|---|
| A1 – DB Bench Press | 10 | 4 | 21X | |
| A2 – BB Pendlay Rows | 15 | - | 21X | |
| B1 - BW Pushups | # | 4 | 21X | |
| B2 – BW Pullups (Or lat pulldowns) | 15 | - | 21X | |
| B3 - Hyper Extensions | 8 | - | 31X | |

## Workout 5 GDW Advanced | Rest: 45 seconds

| Exercise | Reps | Sets | Tempo | Lbs |
|---|---|---|---|---|
| A1 – DB Goblet Squat | 12-15 | 4 | 21X | |

| | | | | |
|---|---|---|---|---|
| A2 – Standing DB Shoulder Press | 8-10 | - | 21X | |
| B1 – BB Deadlift | 8 | 4 | 21X | |
| B2 – Explosive Pushups | # | - | 21X | |
| C1 - Hyper Extensions | 8 | 3 | 31X | |
| C2 – Leg Raises | 8 | - | | |

## Workout 6 IC | Rest: 45 seconds

| Activity | Rest | Duration (s) | Sets | Intensity |
|---|---|---|---|---|
| A1 - Jump Rope | 45 | 60 | 3 | High |
| A2 - Jogging | - | 180 | - | Low |
| B1 - Hill Sprints | 45 | N/A | 4 | High |
| B2 - Jogging | - | 180 | - | Low |

## Workout 7 IC | Rest: 45 seconds

| Activity | Rest | Duration (s) | Sets | Intensity |
|---|---|---|---|---|
| A1 –Incline Treadmill (Or hill sprints) | 45 | 60 | 3 | High |
| A2 – Stationary Bike | - | 180 | - | Low |
| B1 – Jump Rope | 45 | N/A | 4 | High |
| B2 – Treadmill Jog (Or regular jog) | - | 180 | - | Low |

## Workout 8 GDW Circuit| Rest: 90 seconds

| Exercise | Reps | Sets | Tempo | Lbs |
|---|---|---|---|---|
| A1 – BB Squat | # | 3 | 21X | |

| | | | | |
|---|---|---|---|---|
| A2 – BB Deadlift | # | - | 21X | |
| A3 – BB Step Ups | # | - | 21X | |
| A4 – BB Overhead Press | # | - | 21X | |
| A5 – BB Rows | # | - | 31X | |

Blank Workout Templates

**Workout:**          **| Rest:**       **| Day:**

| Exercise | Reps | Sets | Tempo | Lbs |
|----------|------|------|-------|-----|
|          |      |      |       |     |
|          |      |      |       |     |
|          |      |      |       |     |
|          |      |      |       |     |
|          |      |      |       |     |

**Workout:**          | **Rest:**          | **Day:**

| Exercise | Reps | Sets | Tempo | Lbs |
|----------|------|------|-------|-----|
|          |      |      |       |     |
|          |      |      |       |     |
|          |      |      |       |     |
|          |      |      |       |     |
|          |      |      |       |     |

**Workout:**          | **Rest:**          | **Day:**

| Exercise | Reps | Sets | Tempo | Lbs |
|----------|------|------|-------|-----|
|          |      |      |       |     |
|          |      |      |       |     |
|          |      |      |       |     |
|          |      |      |       |     |
|          |      |      |       |     |

# Gift This Book To Someone For Just $1 !

The internet has done a bunch of wonderful, feel good things. No, I'm not talking about easy, unlimited access to porn (though I'm sure that's wonderful in its own right). I'm talking about information in general. There used to be a time where life was simple; a time where your skill, knowledge and influence were your currency. And the beauty of such a currency was that it could never be stolen from you - after all, it was in your head.

Now though, a skill can easily be transferred through the use of multiple mediums. The techniques you read in this book are ones that I currently know to be some the most effective, when it comes to fat loss. If we were in the year 1345, I'd gladly exchange this knowledge in return for bread, meats, fruits, alcohol and/or a sexy maid (what, clean up after myself? Blasphemy!) But in today's world that hardly works, and in order to acquire the things I need, I must rely to the stuff known as *money*.

Look, I can't stop anyone from being an imprudent internet pirate anymore than I can force someone to be a nice little angel, and nor will I bother to. Personally, I don't pay for shit that I don't think is worth my cash, so if that's how you feel, so be it. But when I come across something that has legitimate value, I don't think twice, haggle or bargain. I pay the asking price. I buy nice, so I don't have to buy twice. This has worked out pretty well for me so far.

So if you enjoyed my pull-no-punches rambling and learnt a thing or two that will aid you in your journey to become sexier, then click the button below, and **consider buying a digital copy of this book for someone you care about, for just one dollar!** (The remaining will be billed to you in two easy installments after an entire 14 days). This way they get the book *now*, and you don't have to worry about paying for the book till 2 weeks!

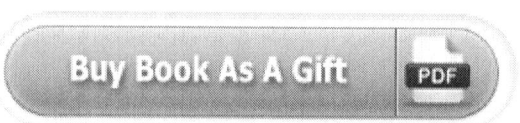

Or use this link: **www.fitjerk.com/giftbook**

**Note:** After your payment goes through, you'll receive a receipt in your inbox from PayPal. Forward this to **info@flawlessfitnessbook.com** along with the gift recipient's name and email. Once you do that, leave the rest to me. I'll tell em' that you bought them the book, how valuable it is (the dollar thing **won't** be mentioned), and why they should be ever so grateful.

Basically, I'll make you look like a glorified angel that shoots shining moonbeams of awesomeness. Trust me, they'll be thanking you for weeks. And honestly, a good book is the best type of present one can get (ok, 2nd to alcohol that is). It's so much better than gift cards – which show you put zero thought into it, and have no taste in general.

"But if I buy this book for my wife or husband, they'll think I'm calling 'em fat!"

Oh relax. You really think that I, the Fittest and Jerkiest of them all would leave you hanging? Any and all objections are handled in the gift email. I've got your ass covered. This will the best dollar you've ever spent on someone.

---

# Notes

# Contents

# CONTENTS

12905703R00131

Printed in Great Britain
by Amazon.co.uk, Ltd.,
Marston Gate.